Fun on Foot in New England

Warwick Ford

with Nola Ford

Wyltan Books
Cambridge, Massachusetts, U.S.A.

ISBN 978-0-9765244-1-0   paperback
ISBN-10: 0-9765244-1-4   paperback
Library of Congress Control Number: 2007920034

Printed in the United States of America by BookMasters, Inc.
Cover Photo: Nola and Warwick at Faneuil Hall, Boston, photo by Louisa Ford
Geographical and street information in maps courtesy the U.S. Geological Survey.

Available in bookstores and online at http://www.funonfoot.com.

Wyltan Books
Cambridge, Massachusetts, U.S.A.

This is a 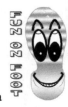 Book

Table of Contents

Preface

The vast majority of us need more exercise. However, many of us struggle with translating that no-brainer into personal action. This observation led to my book *Fun on Foot in America's Cities*. That book was targeted primarily at the frequent traveler who visits different U.S. cities and can use some help and motivation to get outdoors and run, jog, or walk. The main idea was to arm the reader with the information necessary to instantly locate outstandingly pleasant and enjoyable on-foot routes in our largest cities.

Fun on Foot in America's Cities has been a successful title, particularly popular with travelers, ranging from serious marathon runners through to people who just want to get out and walk a good distance. Readers and critics seem to appreciate the overall philosophy and the approach taken in selecting the best on-foot routes in any place.

However, that title is of less value to the person who usually stays near home. Readers based in a particular region would prefer to know more about on-foot routes in their own city or region and less about routes in cities they never visit. The need for more regionally focused adaptations of the Fun-on-Foot model was apparent.

This is the first title in what I plan to be a regional Fun-on-Foot series. I started with New England—the part of the United States that I know best, having been a resident of the region some ten years.

There was a Boston chapter in *Fun on Foot in America's Cities*, featuring five routes close to the city. This book includes all of those routes, but we have had the opportunity to add many more routes in Greater Boston and its surrounds, as well as in other New England populated areas.

The state of urban on-foot trails changes rapidly. Updates to our routes that are brought to our attention will be posted at http://www.funonfoot.com, along with links to other on-line resources useful to the reader. Please visit this site for that information and to share your own local knowledge with the Fun-on-Foot community. We shall also be distributing from that site, for a nominal charge, printer-friendly maps of all routes in this book.

Many people contributed in greater or lesser ways to this book. In our research trips, we talked to innumerable people along the routes and in local bars and coffee shops. Staff of business establishments in the featured centers helped greatly. We also received many ideas by email from local people.

The following individuals stand out for their special help in researching this project or reviewing the manuscript. Geof Newton made particularly valuable contributions to the Cape and the Islands chapter, and we look forward to his own forthcoming book on running in that part of New England. Claude Bench, Elizabeth Lambert, and Tim Smith provided very detailed comments that helped us greatly with the Massachusetts chapters. Marty Schaivone provided valuable ideas on Connecticut. Peter Cressy launched us on the right paths in Vermont. Our good friends Harry and Marcia Greco, who enthusiastically share the Fun-on-Foot philosophy, contributed many ideas. Others who helped in special ways or whose ideas we have used include John Barney, Joe Bator, Jackie Cressy, Lyall Ford, Peter Garrett, Julia Kim, Kevin K. Lynch, Richard Paulsen, Lucy St. John, and Rebecca Wright.

Thank you all for your contributions and for sharing with us your knowledge of and familiarity with your part of the New England region.

I must especially recognize our daughter, Louisa, herself a keen athlete, for her contributions in researching routes, reviewing the manuscript, and providing the cover photo.

Nola and I hope you will enjoy reading and using this book, and that it contributes in some little way to your future quality of life.

Warwick Ford
Cambridge, Massachusetts, U.S.A.

Introduction

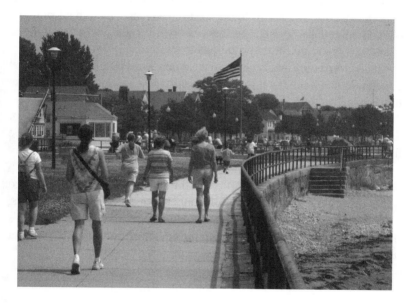

New England is a runner, jogger, walker paradise, with many tremendously enjoyable places to exercise on-foot. If you live in or visit urban New England, this book will help you find the most irresistible outdoor exercise routes. The goal is to remove all barriers to your spending more time outdoors and building fitness while enjoying the region.

The Fun-on-Foot model is a simple one. We (my charming wife and running mate, Nola, and I) are convinced that one of the easiest and most effective ways to keep fit and control weight is to run, jog, or walk in attractive, comfortable, and interesting environments. There are too many excuses for skipping exercise, which is frequently considered a chore, if not downright unpleasant. We believe exercise must be easy and enjoyable if we are to regularly get off our butts.

On-foot exercise—running, jogging, or walking—is an excellent way to keep fit, but doing it in a gym does not pass the ease and enjoyment test (not to mention the budget test) with many people. *Outdoor* on-foot exercise, on the other hand, can definitely be easy and enjoyable. However, one is often unsure of where to go and what will be encountered on the way. Many people hesitate to head out on foot in unfamiliar places because of a shortage of the right information and the absence of a warm fuzzy feeling. All too often, this leads to a convenient excuse for staying indoors or in-vehicle. One must know exactly where to go for that run, jog, or walk.

The information available from websites, local publications, or hotel concierges can help, but it is often out-of-date, rose-tinted, or otherwise unreliable.

We help you get out on-foot by leading you to the very best outdoor exercise places in any location. We always try to be objective. We have a well-defined model for assessing routes, and endeavor to apply a consistent standard everywhere.

This book covers the urban areas in the northeast corner of the United States—the New England states of Connecticut, Maine, Massachusetts, New Hampshire, Rhode Island, and Vermont. We start from the region's metropolis, Boston, and then fan out through the most populous parts of the rest of the region.

* * * *

The Fun-on-Foot books do not generally distinguish between running, jogging, and walking as forms of exercise. While faster exercise builds fitness and burns calories more quickly, all forms are good. On any given outing, Nola and I always start out jogging. If either of our bodies starts to protest loudly enough along the way, we have been known to fall back to walking later. However, we always finish the route. We believe that is most important.

One thing that still surprises me is the number of people who are reluctant to try the routes described in our books saying, "I can't walk four miles, and certainly not ten!" When pressed to try, they almost always retract those preconceptions. Almost anyone without severe disabilities can walk four miles without pain in under an hour-and-a-half and ten miles in three hours or so.

If you are prepared to do some walking but cannot or will not run or jog, this book is still for you. You might be surprised at how rapidly your distances and times improve.

When I say walking, I mean walking at a good pace—not strolling. One of the main impediments we on-foot exercisers face is the person who strolls along at a snail's pace, blocking the sidewalk or pedestrian trail and making no attempt to get his or her blood pumping.

While slow pedestrians are a pain, there is one other entity that really is our Public Enemy Number 1: the *automobile*. The more we can tame our urge to get into that metal box, the more walking, jogging, or running we shall inevitably do. Therefore, when traveling, I do not like renting a car to drive somewhere to run an out-and-back loop from the car park. Since we can often survive and save our precious funds by not renting a car when traveling, I try to exclude automobile dependence throughout our travels in the Fun-on-Foot books.

We generally restrict our route recommendations to the four-to-ten mile range, distances that are not too long for a half-day walk and long enough for a nice run for all but the serious distance runner.

* * * *

In this book, I try to briefly introduce cities or towns to people not familiar with them. However, I give most attention to describing a set of featured routes. Such routes ideally satisfy four attributes: (1) comfort; (2) attractions; (3) convenience; and (4) a destination.

Comfort, which is the most essential attribute, has several elements, all of which are fairly obvious but worth noting. First, there should be minimal safety concerns. There should be a reasonable expectation that there will not be a nasty surprise around the next corner.[1] The number of other people around should be in your comfort zone (not too many and not too few). Underfoot conditions should also be good and there should be a minimum of encounters with vehicular traffic.

---

1   See the table of violent crime statistics for New England cities at the end of this chapter. This table shows that violent crime rates in most of New England are comparatively small, with the only cities exceeding 10 violent crimes per 1,000 inhabitants being: Boston, MA; Bridgeport, CT; Springfield, MA; and Hartford, CT. The figures are from the FBI compilation for 2005.

By *attractions* I mean that the route should be environmentally pleasant and interesting. It helps enormously if a route has points of historic or cultural interest, scenic beauty, or people activities on the day. To be interesting, variety is also highly desirable. Any route can become boring with time, so it is good to have some elements to vary each time. Also, we like to avoid straight out-and-back routes. Repeating everything you saw in the first half of a route on the way back is somehow less satisfying than having something new to see all the way. Therefore, we try to create circular routes; if necessary, we fill in part of the loop by another form of transportation.

Convenience means ease of getting to the start of a route from a city's or town's center or the areas where visitors tend to stay. Similarly, getting back from the end of a route should be easy. Given our belief that the number one enemy of on-foot fitness is the automobile, we try to avoid the need for automobiles in getting to, from, or along our routes. If other forms of transportation are required to close a loop, we look mainly to public transit, so as to minimize costs, hassle, and automobile dependence.

Destination is an important factor to many people but not everyone. Serious runners frequently gain their on-foot satisfaction from successfully meeting their own time and distance goals, and are then content to get straight back to their home or hotel for a shower. However, a lot of people struggle to get out on-foot and to complete a route of sufficient distance. Having a clear destination in mind helps make a route motivating and also reduces the temptation to quit early. If you are mentally on a mission to go somewhere enjoyable, then odds are you will make it there. Therefore, we consider it valuable to have routes end up in places where there is something interesting to see or do afterwards, should one so choose.

Another aspect of a destination that helps many people is having a good food-beverage opportunity waiting at the end. Nola and I have found this works for us. When we first started pushing ourselves to run more, it became apparent that Nola was way more likely to start and complete an eight-mile weekend jog if there was a tasty brunch at the end. I was way more likely to do the same if there was a glass of cold beer at the end.

Is it a bad thing to encourage people to run, jog, or walk to a place where they end up eating and drinking? Won't the damage done by the food and drinks cancel out the good done by the exercise? I think the answer to both questions is, "Not necessarily." You will probably eat anyway. Also, on-foot exercise burns considerable calories (see the table *Estimated Calories Burned in a 5- or 10-mile Route*)[2]. Your calorie-count will end up in much better shape than if you were not exercising at all, giving more leeway for food consumption. Of course, moderation in quantity and wise choice of nutritious foods should always be followed.

Body Weight:	110 lb. (50 Kg.)	150 lb. (68 Kg.)	190 lb. (86 Kg.)
Walking 5 miles	380	500	650
Jogging 5 miles	392	530	674
Running 5 miles	432	567	708
Walking 10 miles	760	1,000	1,300
Jogging 10 miles	783	1,060	1,348
Running 10 miles	864	1,134	1,416

Estimated Calories Burned in a 5- or 10-mile Route
Assumed speeds: Walking 3.0 mph, Jogging 5.2 mph, Running 7.5 mph

Since we believe there is a correlation between the set of people who really relish a good meal or drink and the set of people who most need more exercise, we do not feel anyone should shy away from the food-and-drink motivation angle. A little extra indulgence in the food and drink department is a perfectly reasonable inducement to exercise, especially if you only allow yourself the indulgence if you do the exercise first.

Consequently, one theme you will find in this book is the idea of ending routes near good eating and drinking establishments, where you can wind down if you so choose. We tend to look for pub-restaurants— informal places that will happily accept people in running gear and a little untidy. The eating and drinking part is, of course, entirely

2   Figures computed from data in: Maria Adams, MS, MPH, RD, "The Benefits and Risks of Walking Versus Running," HealthGate http://www. somersetmedicalcenter.com/110324.cfm. Note, however, that calorie burn rate depends on many factors including, but not limited to, amount of skeletal muscle, running efficiency, speed, surface type, incline, resting metabolism, level of fitness, and outside temperature. (Thanks to Ayesha Rollinson for explaining this.) Therefore, consider the figures in the table as indicative only.

optional.   Furthermore, any establishments we mention are purely suggestions from our own experience, and are not intended as exclusive endorsements.

* * * *

New England has many outstanding places to run, jog and walk. There are many scenic routes, thanks to the extensive coastline, river systems, and forested areas (the latter having special appeal in fall). There are also many historic sites that can make an outdoor outing more interesting, especially considering New England's significance as the place of the Pilgrims' first settlment and where the American Revolution started.

The climate throughout the region is also very amenable to outdoor exercise. Our general benchmark for nice outdoor exercise weather is the temperature range 40-to-80 degrees, and New England city averages fall into that range for most of the year (sometimes falling out on the cold side in January and February and out on the warm side in July). Precipitation is limited to roughly one day in three, on average, which is not a major concern.

* * * *

It would not be practical to catalog all nice outdoor routes in New England. What we have done is focus on the major centers of population and the places that most attract visitors. In these places we have sought out the routes that meet our criteria best. In some centers, we found no routes that met our criteria adequately so we omitted those centers from coverage. We have not generally targeted rural areas, so this book makes no pretence to be a New England rural hiking guide.

You might question why we dedicate four chapters to Massachusetts and only one chapter each to the other five states. Given that roughly half the population of New England lives in Massachusetts, we felt this was actually quite reasonable.

We made a point of touring New England extensively and developing our ideas on foot. We tried and rejected many routes that did not meet all criteria. A few routes that we felt were just too good to miss we have flagged as *Fun on Foot Classic Routes*.

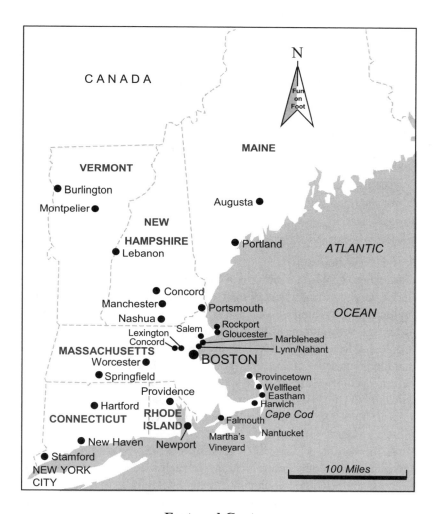

Featured Centers

Some readers will likely enjoy following the exact routes we suggest. However, that is certainly not essential and we expect many of you will take up some of the ideas we present and design your own enjoyable outings around them. In describing our featured routes, we try to provide helpful information for those readers who want to vary the routes with diversions, extensions, or shortcuts.

Since you may not want to carry this book around while out on foot, we have produced a collection of images of the maps of all routes featured, and made that available for download from our website http://www.funonfoot.com for a nominal charge. You can then print your own copy of any map you want, and carry it with you.

If we missed your favorite route, I apologize for that. Please email us your ideas and we shall note them for use in future revisions of this book.

* * * *

One question we often get is what about bikes? Why not cycle these routes? While cycling is a fine fitness activity, we just do not find it very practical when away from home. You are faced with such problems as obtaining a bike, leaving it somewhere safe when you want to go into a restaurant or shop, storing it in the evening, and getting it onto public transit (if that is even possible). Furthermore, we find that many attractive places that are ideal for running or walking do not permit cycling or are just not suitable for cycling. Therefore, while some of our routes use bicycle paths, we do not limit our routes to paths suitable for cycling and, as a consequence, can frequently offer on-footers a superior experience.

Inline skating is closer to on-foot exercise. Some but not all of our routes are suitable for inline skating. In each route description, we try to assess the extent to which inline skating will work.

On that note, let us conclude the lead-in and embark on our tour, focusing on urban on-foot routes with the comfort/attractions/convenience/destination formula as our guiding light. We shall start in Boston, the region's metropolis, and work outward through Massachusetts and then the other New England states.

Our main message: Get out on foot, get fit, see the best of New England, and—most importantly—have fun!

City	Population in 2005	Violent Crimes per 1,000 Inhabitants
Massachusetts		
Boston	567,589	13.17
Cambridge	100,492	4.92
Concord	16,872	1.19
Edgartown	3,929	1.53
Gloucester	30,732	1.53
Lexington	30,335	0.40
Marblehead	20,315	0.10
Nahant	3,610	5.54
Nantucket	10,096	4.06
Newton	83,570	1.36
Provincetown	3,440	6.10
Quincy	89,661	3.78
Salem	41,796	2.34
Springfield	151,670	17.74
Swampscott	14,393	0.49
Waltham	59,068	1.30
Watertown	32,513	1.91
Worcester	175,479	7.92
Connecticut		
Bridgeport	140,177	10.76
Hartford	125,086	11.53
Stamford	120,456	2.95
Maine		
Augusta	18,691	2.19
Portland	64,111	4.16
South Portland	23,589	1.61
New Hampshire		
Concord	42,685	1.62
Lebanon	12,757	1.88
Manchester	110,188	2.80
Nashua	88,113	1.86
Portsmouth	20,953	1.53
Rhode Island		
Newport	25,773	4.27
Providence	177,392	6.80
Vermont		
South Burlington	16,504	1.21

Violent Crime Indexes for New England Cities in 2005

Source: FBI *Crime in the United States* Report 2005

• • • • • • •	Featured on-foot route
· · · · · · · · · ·	Other on-foot routes
——————	Street
— — —	Major highway (No pedestrians)
Ⓣ	MBTA subway or commuter rail station
🚌	Other public transit (Bus, rail, or subway)
🚻	Public restroom
🚻	Public restroom (Seasonal)
🚰	Drinking water
🚰	Drinking water (Seasonal)
🍴	Casual eating/drinking establishment suitable for terminating an athletic route
1	Point of interest
P	Trail parking

Key to Map Symbols

2

Downtown Boston Five-Mile Radius

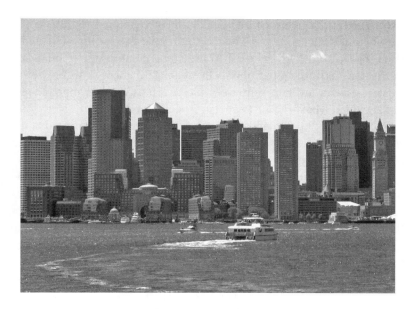

Boston, Massachusetts, is not only the largest city in New England but the heart of a metropolitan area of some four-to-five million inhabitants spanning several municipalities. Since these municipal boundaries are irrelevant to the on-foot exerciser, let me apologize up-front for frequently using the term *Boston* to describe what would more accurately be termed *Greater Boston*.

Boston is a city of the young (the region is host to way more than its fair share of the nation's top colleges) and the young at heart. This makes it a dream city for jogging, running, or walking. There is a massive foot-mobile population, so if you feel like a jog anywhere here you will never feel out of place and rarely be on your own. Do not feel pressured to limit your running to parks or reserves. Running through the streets of downtown Boston or inner suburbs is a perfectly normal activity.

In fact, travel by foot is an important mode of transport in Boston. One reason is the city's compactness, making it easy to negotiate on foot. The more compelling reason, however, is that the traffic system is so dysfunctional many people think twice about driving anywhere in central Boston. The street layout was never planned but grew haphazardly through the roughly 400 years of the region's evolution. The narrowness of the streets has led to many being designated one-way. The result often seems a bewildering navigational nightmare.

The deficiencies in the street system have bred a unique driving style for Boston. Drivers need to use some creativity in getting into traffic streams, turning in front of other vehicles, and so forth. However, Boston drivers are generally very alert, defensive, and more-or-less unflappable. Many out-of-towners (especially people from New York where horn-tooting is mandatory every ten seconds) are amazed at the scarcity of horn tooting in Boston, given the creative driving acts that continually happen.

The driving attitude flows through to pedestrians as well. If you need to cross a busy street, you might have to assert yourself and just cross it. Drivers are generally kind to pedestrians and tend to stop for them without getting particularly upset. (Don't take me too literally on this one, though. You need to develop just the right pedestrian judgment for Boston.)

This type of driving and pedestrian behavior is virtually essential if the people of Boston are to get anywhere at all.

The other alternative to driving is the T—Boston's public transit system that comprises a mixture of subways, buses, commuter trains, and a couple of ferries. The T subway, launched in 1897, was the first U.S. subway system and is the fourth oldest in the world.

The T tends to be somewhat untidy and trashy. Nevertheless, it is convenient, efficient, and generally devoid of the surprises we have encountered in certain other cities' transit systems.

* * * *

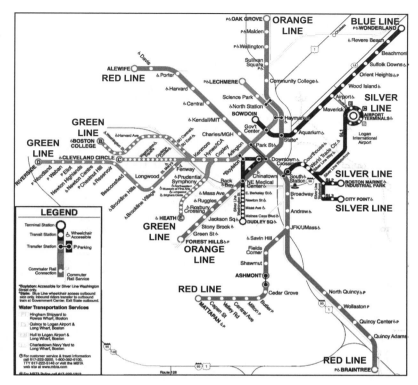

The T Subway System[1]

As to street safety, Boston has a violent crime index of 13 violent crimes per 1,000 inhabitants (in 2005). This is higher than most New England cities but close to the average for large cities nationally. We try to avoid areas with bad reputations, but we must caution you that this matter is ultimately your own responsibility. Please always use good street sense.

* * * *

Now, let us try to pin down the best on-foot exercise routes convenient to central Boston. In this chapter, we cover only routes that are within a five-mile radius of the city center and easily reachable by the T subway. (In the next chapter, we cover routes a little further out.)

There is one no-brainer. The lower Charles River between Boston and Cambridge is one of the best and most popular running, jogging,

---

1   Grayscale adaptation of map provided by the copyright holder, MBTA.

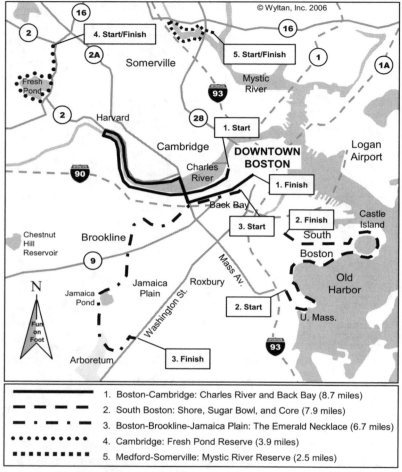

1. Boston-Cambridge: Charles River and Back Bay (8.7 miles)
2. South Boston: Shore, Sugar Bowl, and Core (7.9 miles)
3. Boston-Brookline-Jamaica Plain: The Emerald Necklace (6.7 miles)
4. Cambridge: Fresh Pond Reserve (3.9 miles)
5. Medford-Somerville: Mystic River Reserve (2.5 miles)

Featured Routes in Five-Mile Radius of Downtown Boston

and walking areas in the country. We have built our first route there, linking up with some of Boston's most historical precincts. After that, we have selected some other routes that take in South Boston and the ocean shore, the Emerald Necklace to Jamaica Plain, Fresh Pond in Cambridge, and the Mystic River Reserve, north of downtown. We believe we have nailed the best routes conveniently accessible from downtown.

Boston-Cambridge: Charles River and Back Bay

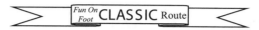

Distance	8.7 miles (or 4.4 miles; or other variants)
Comfort	Excellent running conditions. Plenty of on-foot exercisers around. Crowds are unlikely to be a concern unless you hit a special event. OK for inline skating.
Attractions	Pass by or near several city sights, including the Hatch Shell, MIT, Harvard University, Trinity Church, and the old Granary Burial Ground. Most of the route follows a very pleasant riverside pedestrian/bicycle trail and the rest is along wide, runner-friendly streets.
Convenience	Start at the T Red Line Charles/MGH station, a short walk or T ride from anywhere in downtown Boston or Cambridge. End at the Boston Common, close to downtown shops, the financial district, theatre district, Copley Place, Hynes Convention Center, and the T Red Line Park station. Alternatively, the 4.4 mile shortened route ends near the T Red Line Harvard station.
Destination	Boston Common, the launch point for Boston's historic Freedom Trail, near downtown shops and some excellent restaurants and pubs for winding down. The 4.4-mile variation ends at lively Harvard Square, the center of the Harvard community, with shops, restaurants, and pubs.

Our first route centers on the Charles River, combined with Back Bay. This is one of our hometown favorite routes. It scores high on all the attributes of comfort, attractions, convenience, and destination. While we describe one particular eight-mile route, you can vary it in many ways to better fit your personal tastes.

This route uses the Dr. Paul Dudley White Bicycle Path, a loop stretching from the Science Museum upstream nine miles to Watertown on both sides of the Charles River. It is (very appropriately) dedicated to the "Father of Modern Cardiology," one of Boston's famous sons (1886-1973).

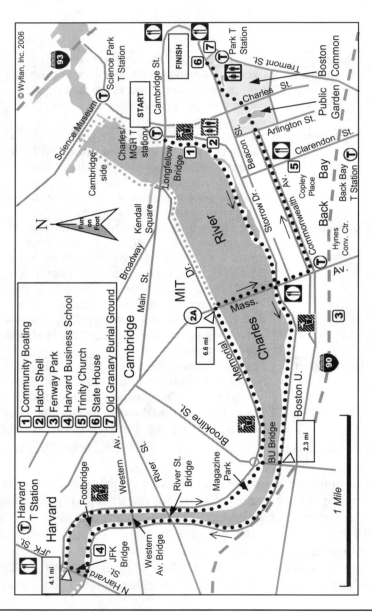

The whole route is paved. However, for much of its length you will find well-traveled dirt side paths or grassy verges that make it very runner-friendly. Restroom facilities are scarce; in fact the only one is at the Hatch Shell. There are a few water fountains but they are disabled from late fall through early spring.

Our route starts at the Boston end of the Longfellow Bridge, named after Henry Wadsworth Longfellow, Maine-born, but generally considered one of Boston's favorite sons. This spot is not far from hotels in downtown Boston and eastern Cambridge. If you are not within walking distance, take the T Red Line to the Charles/MGH station.

Cross the footbridge to the riverbank and then head upstream on the Boston side of the river. The other side of the river is all part of Cambridge, with its diverse community of students, academics, and others.

Pass Community Boating, where Bostonians (Nola and I included) learn to sail. The swirling winds in the Charles Basin, coming off the nearby downtown high-rises, present ever variable, challenging, and fun sailing conditions. The objective is to venture forth in a 15-foot centerboard boat and avoid getting dunked in the dirty Charles.[2]

The riverside path then takes you through Boston's best-known outdoor recreational area, the Esplanade. This nicely landscaped park is home to many community events.

Pass the Edward M. Hatch Memorial Shell, a major outdoor entertainment site, and the center of such outstanding events as the July 4th fireworks to the accompaniment of the Boston Pops. This is also where many organized runs and walks start or end. On the opposite bank of the Charles is Massachusetts Institute of Technology (MIT), the world-leading engineering and science school.

Cross the footbridge and pass the sculpture of Arthur Fiedler, renowned and beloved conductor of the Boston Pops for fifty years.

Continuing up the river, at 1.2 miles from the Longfellow Bridge is the next bridge, whose name is a source of some confusion. It is officially named the Harvard Bridge, having been dedicated to Reverend John Harvard. Unfortunately, it is nowhere near Harvard University. In fact, its Cambridge endpoint is right in the middle of MIT, so some people call it the MIT Bridge. Because the road it carries is Mass. Av. (you

---

2   A visitor can buy a part-year membership of Community Boating or just walk in with the hope of hitching a free joyride with a local sailor.

would never, ever speak out the full "Massachusetts Avenue" words in Boston), we shall call it the Mass. Av. Bridge. This is the name most locals will instantly understand.

While you have various route choices at this point, we suggest continuing upstream on the Boston side.

The stretch up to the Boston University (BU) Bridge is particularly pleasant. The buildings on the Boston side here are part of Boston University, the fourth largest independent university in the United States. The pedestrian path takes you under the BU Bridge on a short boardwalk. This is not the most convenient place to cross the river. If you need to do that, first cross Storrow Drive via the pedestrian overpass downstream from the river bridge, and then follow sidewalks around BU up to the river bridge.

The conditions after the BU Bridge are less than perfect, comprising mainly a paved bicycle path adjacent to busy Storrow Drive. However, the scenery along the river is still pleasant. Roughly a mile from the BU Bridge is the River Street Bridge, the first place you need to stop for cars. Cross River Street at the pedestrian crossing. At this point, you could cross the river and head back downstream, but our featured route continues upstream.

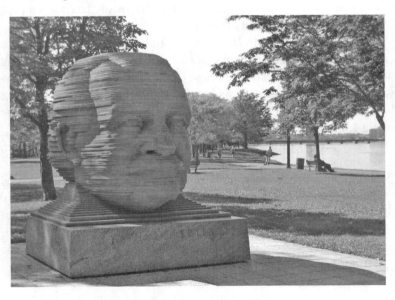

Arthur Fiedler Listens for the Sound of the Pops

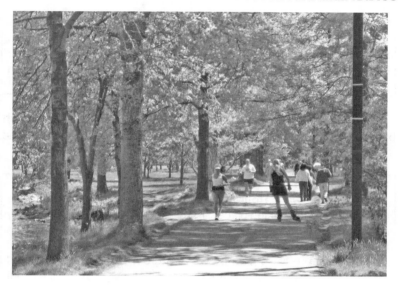

Charles River Trail Near the Esplanade

The Western Avenue Bridge is a quarter mile from the River Street Bridge. Cross Western Avenue. You now enter Harvard territory and conditions improve greatly in all respects. Harvard University, established in 1636, claims to be the first college established in North America. Continuing upstream, as you approach the Harvard footbridge (more correctly the John W. Weeks pedestrian bridge), you see on your left the Harvard Business School. This is where Lou Gerstner, Michael Bloomberg, and George W. Bush obtained their MBAs—whereas, across the river, Bill Gates dropped out of his undergraduate program as a junior. (If you ever become bored running, there lies a fertile topic for contemplation.)

Cross the river at the next bridge, which links the Allston and Cambridge campuses of Harvard. This bridge is formally named the Larz Anderson Bridge, in recognition of a local political and diplomatic figure (1866-1937). However, locals will more likely recognize it as the JFK Bridge since, on the Cambridge side, it feeds JFK Street at JFK Memorial Park.

> **VARIATION**
>
> If you want to extend our route by two miles, continue upstream roughly a mile and cross the river at the Eliot Bridge. There is a water fountain there, and on-foot conditions are good throughout. Then continue back downstream to Harvard on the Cambridge side.

At the Cambridge end of the JFK Bridge, you are just a few short blocks from Harvard Square, the center of the Harvard campus and community.

> **VARIATION**
>
> If you only want a four-mile outing, you can stop here. There are many eating and drinking places, ranging from student joints to quality restaurants. For the on-footer we can recommend: John Harvard's Brewery (Dunster Street, one block east of JFK Street near Mount Auburn Street, with its own brews and great food); Legal Seafood at the Charles Hotel (Eliot Street, one block west of JFK, with great seafood and a casual bar/bistro atmosphere); and Grendel's Den (on the left side of JFK Street at Winthrop Street, a down-home pub for all ages with a wide selection of inexpensive food). You can then explore the Harvard campus and the nearby bookstores and museums. Return to downtown Boston via the T Red Line from Harvard Station at the north end of JFK Street.

From the Cambridge end of the JFK Bridge, head downstream on the Cambridge side of the Charles following Memorial Drive. It is 2.5 miles back to the Mass. Av. Bridge. The stretch from Harvard past the footbridge to the Western Avenue Bridge is particularly pleasant on Sundays from mid-spring to mid-fall, since Memorial Drive is closed to traffic. After that you pass the River Street Bridge. You then pass Magazine Park and come to a large rotary with an overpass for Memorial Drive traffic. Keep hard right and pass the Cambridge end of the BU Bridge. Don't cross that bridge. Rather, continue downstream on the paved sidewalk across the rail tracks. Note that the steps down towards the river here lead to a dead-end.

You will probably notice considerable bird life along the river, especially Canada Geese and ducks. However, here near the BU Bridge there is a different bird-life family—a flock of 60-plus white geese that live year-round here. Most members of the local community either love or despise these birds.

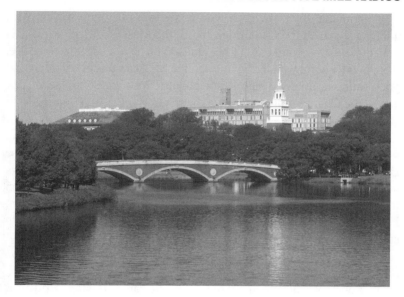

The Charles River at Harvard

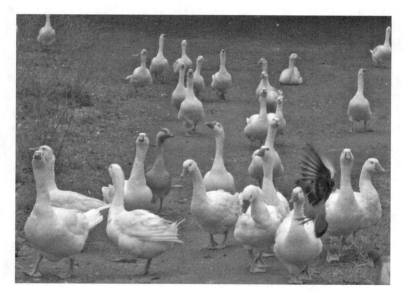

The Cambridge White Geese Greet Visitors

Continuing down the river, you come to a busy intersection with a traffic signal, at the Cambridge end of the Mass. Av. Bridge. This is very close to the center of MIT but, unless you have a specific objective, there is little point wandering through the MIT campus or trying to find good eating or drinking places thereabouts. We suggest you head back across the Charles at this point via the Mass. Av. Bridge (Route 2A) to Back Bay.

Back Bay is a rare exception to Boston's confusing streets tradition, with its streets following an organized rectangular grid. This is because Back Bay did not even exist until the mid-1800s, when the city's leaders launched an ambitious 30-year program to landfill the marshlands on the south bank of the Charles River adjacent to downtown. Navigating Back Bay is made even easier by knowing that the main north-south streets are named with their leading letters in alphabetical order—starting from the east, Arlington Street, Berkeley Street, Clarendon Street, and so on.

Our on-foot route continues to the historic part of Boston. However, if you wanted to stop earlier, you will find a range of good eating and drinking places throughout Back Bay. The first encountered that we like is the Crossroads Pub, an Irish pub on Beacon Street 50 yards west of Mass. Av. This place claims to be Back Bay's oldest pub, established immediately at the end of prohibition.

To continue, keep on Mass. Av. to the third light, then take a left along the center path of the Commonwealth Avenue Mall. This is a beautiful street—a 100-foot wide strip with generous pedestrian space, light vehicle traffic, and magnificent buildings on both sides. The buildings were constructed in the latter half of the nineteenth century as Back Bay evolved through the filling-in of the marshlands. Originally these buildings were single-family residences. In the twentieth century, many were converted to condominiums or commercial use, but the overall external architecture and atmosphere have been preserved largely intact.

You will encounter several interesting statues and memorials along this eight-block route. For example, the Boston Women's Memorial recognizes three of Boston's famous daughters—Abigail Adams, Lucy Stone, and Phillis Wheatley—who, through their writings, made major contributions to social change.

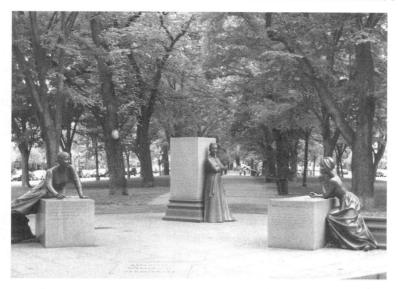

Commonwealth Avenue Trail and the Boston Women's Memorial

You cross several lightly trafficked streets. You might consider ending your route at Clarendon Street since, if you turn right here, you come to one of Back Bay's most famous buildings, Trinity Church, consecrated in 1876. The history of efforts to keep this entire beautiful establishment above the water level makes interesting reading. Also, across Clarendon Street from Trinity Church, there is a great seafood restaurant that is our top recommendation for Sunday Brunch in this part of Boston. Skipjack's excellent Sunday seafood brunch includes a jazz accompaniment. It is a teensy bit up-market, so bear that in mind when launching into here in your running gear. However, it has a bar area that comfortably accommodates all comers.

To continue to the end of our route, keep on Commonwealth Avenue to its termination at Arlington Street and the Boston Public Garden. Cross Arlington Street and enter the garden, passing Washington's statue. Cycling and inline skating are not permitted in the garden, but all forms of on-foot exercise are. Cross the footbridge over the swan boat rides. Continue straight through the garden to Charles Street and cross that street.

You then enter Boston Common, America's first public park, established in 1634. The Public Garden and Boston Common are lovely places for wandering and people watching but not a great running environment because of the crowds. Therefore, consider this a nice wind-down stretch.

Take the left path, northeastward through the Boston Common to Beacon Street. Continue to the Massachusetts State House, whose gold-leaf dome you cannot miss. This point, the nominal end point of our route, is also the start of Boston's Freedom Trail, the red sidewalk-marked trail that leads you through Boston's most famous historic sites.

Although Nola and I have run the Freedom Trail a couple of times, we do not recommend that because of the many slow tourists and the temptation to stop and look at things yourself. You might as well consider it a sightseeing walk. To get started, follow Park Street to Tremont Street (Boston's original name was Tremontaine, reflecting the three hills that once dominated the landscape here). Turn left into Tremont Street and you come to the first major Freedom Trail site—the Old Granary Burial Ground, where Samuel Adams, John Hancock, and Paul Revere rest. Then follow the red line to complete the Freedom Trail experience.

If you are ready for a food or drink break, there are many good establishments around here. We can recommend two top-class Irish pub/restaurants nearby. The first is Emmett's, a little further along Beacon Street from the State House, near Tremont Street. The food and décor are excellent and brunch is served on Saturday and Sunday.

For our other recommendation, head north on Tremont Street, which leads into Cambridge Street. Across from City Hall on Cambridge Street is the Kinsale Irish Pub & Restaurant, which has a genuine Celtic décor, good food and beer, and entertainment most evenings and for Sunday brunch.

Some other major Freedom Trail attractions are nearby. The Old State House is on State Street, off Cambridge Street near City Hall. Faneuil Hall (which, for the enlightenment of our French-speaking Canadian compatriots, is pronounced *fan-yull* hall) is just north of City Hall. Recognized as America's *Cradle of Liberty*, Faneuil Hall served as a central location for organizing protests against the British prior to the Revolution.

There are several other notable pub/restaurants nearby on the Freedom Trail. They include the Bell in Hand, which claims to be the oldest tavern in the country, with a history back to 1795, and the Union Oyster House, the oldest restaurant in Boston, established in 1826 in a building with a history back to 1742.

There are many more historic sites near here, and tacking some more sedate tourist activities onto the end of a good Charles River and Back Bay run, jog, or walk can mean an enormously satisfying day.

* * * *

You will realize by now that, given the presence of trails on both sides of the Charles River and the number of bridges, you can construct many different routes of varying length along the Charles. The following graphic gives component mileages, allowing you to calculate lengths of routes you might devise.

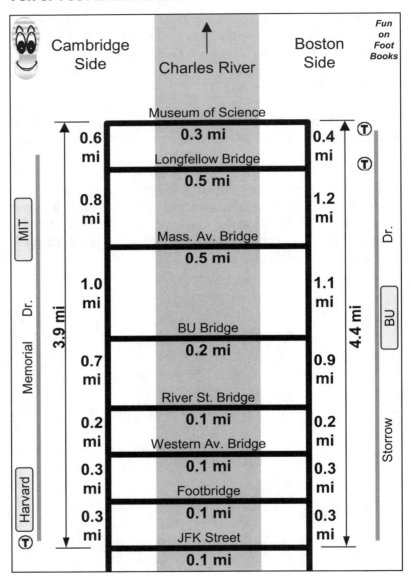

Lower Charles River Mileages

South Boston: Shore, Sugar Bowl, and Core

Distance	7.9 miles
Comfort	Excellent on-foot conditions along an oceanfront trail for most of the route, with plenty of pedestrians around and few encounters with vehicle cross-traffic. The first half-mile and final mile-and-a-half are along street sidewalks. Crowds are unlikely to be a concern. Mostly but not entirely suitable for inline skating.
Attractions	A beautiful seaside trail, passing popular beaches, the U. Mass. Campus, the JFK Library and Museum, and Castle Island/Fort Independence. Touch the pulse of Boston's most famous Irish community residential area.
Convenience	Start and end at T stations on the Red Line, which provides direct service to the financial district, downtown shops, theatre district, Cambridge, and southeastern Boston suburbs. Alternatively, at the end, you can walk to the Seaport Hotel or the World Trade Center area, or catch a bus downtown.
Destination	Several excellent Irish pub/restaurants in South Boston.

If you like seashore routes, this is Boston's best, with close to six miles of gorgeous trails along the water. Making it more interesting, it centers on *Southie*, the number one residential area for Boston's Irish community.

Take the T Red Line to the JFK/U Mass station and follow the signs "To Buses." Once outside, bear right and pass the bus area. There is a three-way road intersection here with a traffic signal. Pick up the street sidewalk of the rightmost road, Morrissey Boulevard, heading south towards the supermarket. At the supermarket, take the footbridge over the road.

Continue south on the other side of the road, past the Boston College High School, to the main entrance road to the University of Massachusetts at Boston. Cross that road and pick up the paved pedestrian trail to the left, heading east along the waterfront. This is a

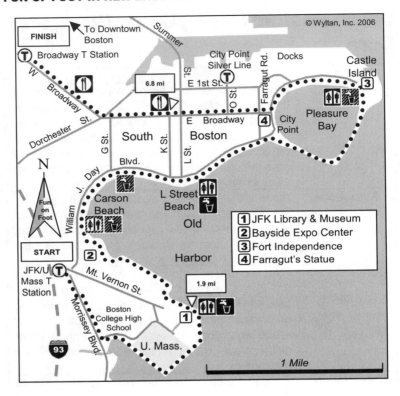

very pleasant trail, far away from automobiles and with plenty of fresh ocean air. Follow the water around until you come to the JFK Library and Museum.

The JFK Library and Museum portrays the life and legacy of President Kennedy. Highlights include the family gallery of photographs and film coverage of the debate between John Kennedy and Richard Nixon in the 1960 presidential election campaign, the Cuban Missile Crisis, Walter Cronkite's announcement of the President's assassination, and the funeral. You probably do not want to interrupt your on-foot exercise at this early stage, but you might wish to come back here later.

Continue north and west on the coastal trail around the edge of the bay known variously as Old Harbor or Dorchester Bay. A short part of the trail is unsealed. On the opposite side of the bay is South Boston, your end destination. Just over a mile from the JFK library you come to Carson Beach, a popular local destination on hot summer days. From

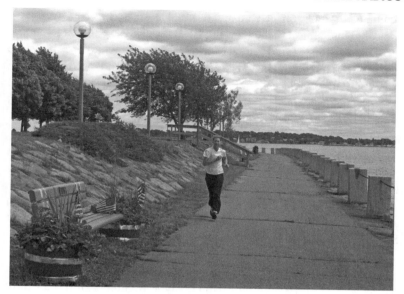

The Ocean Trail by U. Mass.

that point on, follow beach frontage to City Point, where the beach ends and a small collection of yacht clubs takes over the waterfront.

At this point you enter an interesting area known as Castle Island or "the sugar bowl." It comprises a large tidal pool (called Pleasure Bay), fully enclosed by a manmade causeway. Go completely around the causeway (roughly 1.6 miles). If the wind is right, you might be entertained (or annoyed) by low flying jet aircraft, landing or taking off at nearby Logan Airport.

At the northeast corner of the causeway you encounter Fort Independence, on what was once a small island. This site has hosted various forts since 1634, all known at their time as "The Castle." The present edifice dates back to 1851 and played an active military role right through World Wars I and II. Guided tours operate on Saturday and Sunday afternoons, June through August, and Sundays in September and October.

Continue following the paved trail from the fort, westward around Pleasure Bay, until you encounter a statue of Admiral David Farragut located somewhat haphazardly in the middle of the road. The U.S. Navy's first admiral has stood here for over a hundred years, wistfully scanning the horizon in vain for the first glimpse of a tall warship's topsail. This statue and the Pleasure Bay causeway are all that remain of an 1890's vision to build a great Marine Park here, including a showcase aquarium. The South Boston Aquarium was built and did operate here from 1912 until 1954, when the whole venture tanked (pardon the pun) through lack of funds. The building was then razed. Now, this area contains a lovely beach, sporting, and recreation area—one of the best-kept locals' secrets.

Farragut's statue marks the eastern extremity of Broadway, the main thoroughfare threading South Boston end-to-end, and the road to follow to conclude this route.

South Boston is a famous and historical part of Boston, best known as the home of a large community of Irish immigrants. It follows that South Boston is also home to many Irish pubs, therefore an ideal place to end a nice day out on-foot.

The quality of South Boston's pubs varies widely. We like, in particular, the Playwright on E Broadway at K Street. It has a hearty atmosphere, a comprehensive food menu, and brunch on Saturday and Sunday. Running gear and non-locals are always welcome.

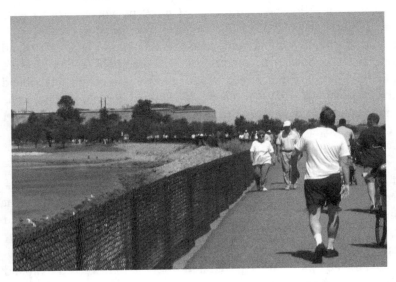

The Pedestrian Causeway at Castle Island, Approaching Fort Independence

VARIATION

If you want to get back to the Seaport Hotel or World Trade Center area from near the Playwright, take L Street north from E Broadway. It leads straight to Summer Street in the middle of that part of the city.

Another good pub/restaurant choice is Shenannigans on W Broadway half a mile beyond the Playwright.

To get back to downtown Boston from either of these pubs, the most reliable way is to follow Broadway to the T Red Line Broadway station, which is 1.1 miles from the Playwright. Other alternatives are a bus service in L Street to downtown via Summer Street, or a T Silver Line service from O Street and 1st Street, but check service schedules for both in advance, especially on weekends.

Boston-Brookline-Jamaica Plain: The Emerald Necklace

Distance	6.7 miles
Comfort	Mostly excellent on-foot conditions under shady trees. There is some need to cross and follow trafficked streets. Expect a number of other on-foot exercisers around but crowds are unlikely to be a concern. Not generally suitable for inline skating.
Attractions	Experience some very attractively landscaped parks and trails close to central Boston. Escape completely from the bustle and the traffic in some parts.
Convenience	Start near the Public Garden, handy to T Red and Green Line stations and hotels in the financial district, theatre district, Copley Place, or Hynes Convention Center vicinity. End at the T Orange Line Green Street station. The Orange line takes you direct to Back Bay, the Hynes Convention Center, Copley Place, the theatre district, the financial district, and northern suburbs.
Destination	Doyle's Café, one of Boston's most famous Irish establishments for eating, drinking, and carousing.

The Emerald Necklace extends from Back Bay to Jamaica Plain. Frederick Law Olmsted, designer of New York's Central Park, created the Emerald Necklace circa 1875. The overall plan involved a string of nine arguably contiguous "parks" stretching roughly eight miles in all. We have already covered the first three of these "parks"—the Boston Common, the Public Garden, and Commonwealth Avenue Mall—all of which predated Olmsted.

Olmsted's plan tacked on a string of further parks, following the course of the Muddy River, a stream feeding the Charles River. The Muddy River was long an embarrassment to Boston's inhabitants— a smelly, marshy annoyance. One of Olmsted's missions was to hide the Muddy River. He largely succeeded with that, although its unpleasantness still shows through when you get close enough at various spots today.

Heading progressively upstream, Olmsted's parks include the Back Bay Fens, the Riverway, Olmsted Park, Jamaica Pond, the Arnold Arboretum, and Franklin Park.

Running the course of these Muddy River parks is generally very pleasant; although you will need to cross a few busy roads *en route*. Our featured route only goes as far as the Arboretum, leaving Franklin Park to the more adventurous.

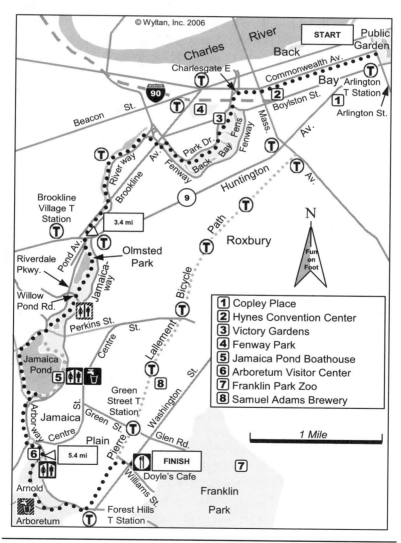

© Wyltan, Inc. 2006

1 Copley Place
2 Hynes Convention Center
3 Victory Gardens
4 Fenway Park
5 Jamaica Pond Boathouse
6 Arboretum Visitor Center
7 Franklin Park Zoo
8 Samuel Adams Brewery

Start at Commonwealth Avenue and Arlington Street in Back Bay, near the Public Garden. You can easily get here from the T Red Line Park station or Green Line Arlington station. Alternatively, if you are staying near Copley Place or the Hynes Convention Center, take the nearest northbound street up to Commonwealth Avenue.

Follow Commonwealth Avenue westbound, backtracking what we described in our first route. Cross Mass. Av., avoiding the underpass and keeping to the left, or southern, sidewalk. At Charlesgate E, turn left and take the sidewalk up the road ramp that emerges here. Go over Interstate 90 and cross Boylston Street at the light at the top of the ramp. You see Fenway Park, home of the Red Sox, away on your right. You also come to a sign announcing the start of the Back Bay Fens.

Enter the park and find yourself amidst a very impressive collection of community gardens. The centerpiece of this area is the Richard D. Parker Memorial Victory Garden. These gardens represent the last remaining of the region's victory gardens created during World War II. At that time, demands for food exports to the nation's armed forces in Europe and the Pacific caused rationing and shortages for those back home in the States. In response, President Roosevelt called for Americans to grow more vegetables. The City of Boston established 49 areas (including the Boston Common and the Public Gardens) as "victory gardens" for citizens to grow vegetables and herbs.

Today, these gardens are something special. Most are nurtured for their natural beauty more so than for bearing vegetables or flowers to cut and take away. Local individuals and families spend countless hours creating their own decorative piece of a remarkable landscape. There are various routes through the Back Bay Fens and their gardens, so take your pick.

The area is bounded on the left by the street called simply "Fenway" and on the right by Park Drive. As you emerge from the Fens area you find yourself on one of these streets, which lead to a very complicated intersection involving both Boylston Street and Brookline Avenue.

This "intersection" is a traffic nightmare for drivers, let alone us poor pedestrians. You need to cross the intersection in a generally northerly direction from where the Fens end. We recommend getting to the left, or outermost, side of Fenway before or at the first traffic signal. Cross Brookline Avenue and follow Fenway's left side into the bend where it changes name to Riverway. Cross the street at the marked pedestrian crossing. The main advice is to avoid getting into the center traffic island areas after Brookline Avenue since, despite the existence of pedestrian crossings; it is hard to get safely to where you want to go.

Sanity returns when you find the trailhead and sign welcoming you to the Riverway.

Along the Riverway, on-foot conditions are excellent. There are trails along both sides of the watercourse. We prefer the left (southeastern) side, which is unpaved and generally devoid of cyclists who prefer the other side that is paved. The left side is also further away from the sometimes-invasive T Green Line. You are treated to various interesting environmental enhancements, such as stone bridges and other structures, thanks to Mr. Olmsted's artistic ingenuity.

The first busy street you need to cross is Brookline Avenue. After crossing it, bear right following the tree-lined trail along its south side. Continue past Brookline Ice & Coal to where Brookline intersects Route 9. Cross Route 9 at the light. On the south side of Route 9, head back east a couple of hundred yards and find Pond Street and the sign welcoming you to Olmsted Park.

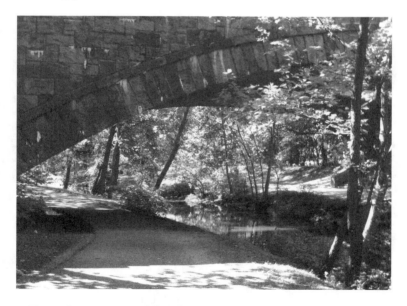

The Riverway Trail and an Example of Olmsted's Stone Bridge Structures

Olmsted Park has nicely varied terrain, with its share of wilderness areas and attractive landscaping. There are various ways through the park. You can bear right and follow a paved trail. This trail splits into separate pedestrian and bicycle tracks for much of the way. Alternatively, if you start off bearing left, you can pick up an unpaved trail through the middle of the park. This trail and a little network of dirt paths that link to it are particularly pleasant since they give you complete escape from traffic and most of the people. Yet another alternative is to keep bearing hard left, where there is a paved path following Jamaicaway down the east edge of the park.

Whichever path you choose, proceed south to Willow Pond Road, cross it and continue south to Perkins Street. Cross Perkins Street and you come to Jamaica Pond—a large, circular and very picturesque pond, with a 1.4-mile pedestrian path around it. You can go around the pond either way. The more attractive option is to bear to the right, and go around the pond counterclockwise. However, if you need to use facilities, go the clockwise direction— this takes you past the Jamaica Pond Boat House where there are restrooms and a water fountain.

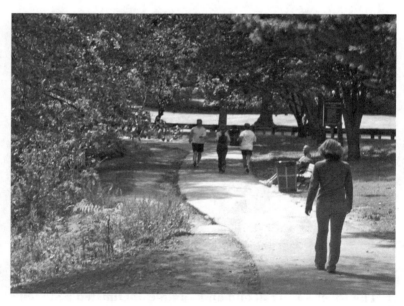

The Trail Around Jamaica Pond

Continue to the south end of the lake where you see a road curving off towards the southwest, as part of a larger system of roads to the south. This is Arborway, the road system connecting Jamaica Pond and the Arnold Arboretum. Take the right hand sidewalk along Arborway to a large rotary, admiring the charming houses along the way. Follow the edge of the rotary around to the right, crossing Centre Street (yes, it really is spelt that way). Despite the marked pedestrian crossing adjacent to the rotary, you might find it difficult crossing here; if so, go 100 yards up Centre Street and cross at the light.

Now follow the road around to the southeast away from the rotary (the road is still called Arborway here, or Route 203). After a short distance, you come to the main entrance to the Arboretum.

Vehicles are generally excluded from the Arboretum, so it is a pedestrian's delight. There are wide roads and paths to follow, with plenty of room for runners, joggers, walkers, and plant gazers alike. Admission is free.

Inside this entrance to the right is the Hunnewell Building, housing a Visitor Center. Except on holidays, you can obtain a map and information here and use the restrooms.

VARIATIONS

There are some excellent trails within the Arboretum, which we do not detail here. Most notably there are two big hills with scenic but different views. Peters Hill is a strenuous climb that rewards you with an excellent view of downtown Boston from the top. Bussey Hill has a view towards the peaceful southwest.

Our featured route proceeds through the Arboretum, along Meadow Road. Pass the maple tree area and come to the three picturesque ponds designed by Olmsted. Turn left into Forest Hills Road. Exit the Arboretum via the Forest Hills gate. Turn right along the Arborway and follow the road down the exit ramp to the Forest Hills T station.

Continuing on from the T station, cross Route 203 at the light. Here you find a sign welcoming you to the Pierre Lallement bicycle path. This path is dedicated in memory of the French gentleman who is attributed with "inventing the bicycle." (I sometimes fantasize what it might have been like to be a neighbor of someone inventing the bicycle, observing it from your window...)

The Pierre Lallement trail, also known as the Southwest Corridor Linear Park, follows the route of the T Orange Line above the ground right back to Back Bay. We are not going that far though. Take the trail past the first bridge over the T tracks then bear right into Williams Street past the English High School. Follow Williams Street one block to Washington Street where there is a special restaurant/pub destination.

F.J. Doyle's Braddock Café is one of the most famous eating and drinking places in Boston, and a worthy on-foot destination for anyone who enjoys food, beer, single-malt scotches, or just a great pub environment. Doyle's, which opened in 1882, has been a center of Irish political life back to the days of John F. Fitzgerald, the first Irish-American to become Mayor of Boston. It is frequented by such well-known folk as Senator John Kerry and Boston Mayor Tom Menino. There are photos celebrating visits by President Bill Clinton and Senator Edward Kennedy (who dedicated the John F. Fitzgerald Room in memory of his late grandfather in 1988). Photos of Presidents Jack Kennedy and Franklin D. Roosevelt are also prominent. Breakfast is served every day, brunch is offered on Saturdays and Sundays, and you

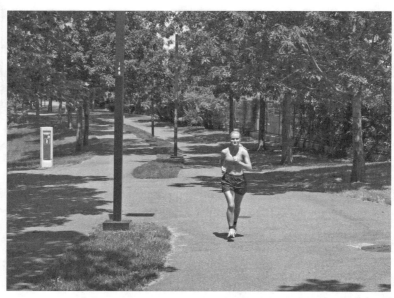

The Lallement Trail near its Arboretum End

can expect a good time. One little caution: Doyle's does not accept credit cards.

After enough chatting with the locals at Doyle's, you can return to central Boston via the T Orange Line. Go back up Williams Street to the T line and Lallement trail, turn right along Amory Street, and find the Green Street station two blocks further on.

Franklin Park, with 15 miles of pedestrian paths, is another place to run near here. Turn right on Green Street. After crossing Washington Street it becomes Glen Road, which leads to Franklin Park. While Franklin Park once did not have a very good reputation, it has been substantially improved over the past several years. You might also visit the Franklin Park Zoo.

The Samuel Adams Brewery is nearby and afternoon tours are offered some days of the week. To get to the brewery, continue north along the T line past Green Street a few short blocks to Porter Street. The brewery is on Porter Street.

If you are still feeling energetic, you can take the Lallement trail on-foot back to Back Bay. We are disinclined to recommend that, however, as its surrounds are quite uninspiring.

Cambridge: Fresh Pond Reserve

Distance	3.9 miles
Comfort	There is a 0.7-mile trek along street sidewalks and park access paths to and from the Fresh pond trail, which is a 2.5-mile paved pedestrian-only loop. Expect plenty of other pedestrians, many with dogs. Not suitable for inline skating in parts.
Attractions	A very scenic trail around a reservoir, with natural parkland all around and some wildlife. While being in a highly urban area, this trail provides excellent (and often welcome) escape from automobile traffic and the bustle of the city.
Convenience	Start and end at Alewife station on the T Red Line, roughly four miles west of downtown Boston. The Red Line provides direct service to the financial district, downtown shops, the theatre district, Cambridge, and southeastern Boston suburbs.
Destination	The Alewife Brook Parkway area on Cambridge's west boundary. There are shops and several wind-down restaurants and bars here.

This short route is very popular with Cambridge locals but can also be easily reached via the T from downtown Boston or anywhere else on the Red Line. What makes it special is its escape from the automobile scene, an attraction that the lower Charles River just cannot offer.

Take the T Red Line to Alewife. Follow the exit signs pointing to Cambridgepark Drive. Go past the big silver T sign and cross Cambridgepark Drive. Then bear left along the paved footpath that becomes the sidewalk of the Alewife Brook Parkway. Proceed to the rotary, passing Fresh Pond Mall. Bear right up Concord Avenue and cross that street at the pedestrian light. Go straight into Fresh Pond Reserve and pick up the paved trail around the reservoir. This is a very pleasant trail, popular with local walkers and joggers. The distance around the reservoir is 2.5 miles.

Assume you go clockwise around. You pass the Cambridge Water Works, which has public facilities when open. Further south, the trail forks with a paved trail to the left and a small, unpaved trail to the right. The unpaved trail can be questionable if there has been recent rain, so we suggest you avoid that. You then come to a fork of paved trails, and we recommend the right-hand choice, which takes you close to the water around Kingsley Park.

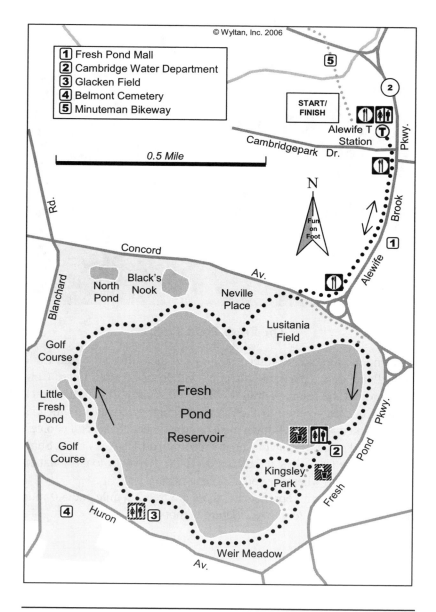

VARIATION
Take the left-hand branch and bypass Kingsley Park, cutting the distance by 0.25 mile.

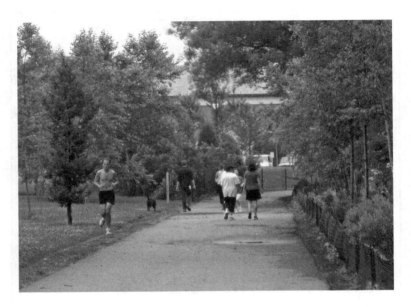

The Fresh Pond Trail

Continue around the reservoir, passing the golf course and Little Fresh Pond, a very pleasant little pond with loads of water lilies. Continue around the reservoir trail to where you started it, and backtrack across Concord Avenue to the Alewife Brook Parkway commercial area. If you want a wind-down meal or drink, there are several choices. For a casual place, we can personally recommend Tin Alley Grill, Summer Shack, or Bertucci's at the Alewife T. Proceed back to the T station and ride the T to wherever you are going next.

For the competitively inclined, there are free 2.5-mile and 5.0-mile races around Fresh Pond every Saturday morning.

Medford-Somerville: Mystic River Reserve

Distance	2.5 miles
Comfort	This is a generally nice loop on dedicated pedestrian/bicycle trails, good underfoot, away from traffic in some parts but close to noisy roads in other parts. Expect other pedestrians around. Not suitable for inline skating in parts.
Attractions	Quite scenic in parts, traversing natural parkland. While being in the middle of a highly urban area and close to Interstate 93, this trail provides a good opportunity for on-foot exercise without direct traffic encounters.
Convenience	Start and end at Station Landing or the Wellington Circle station on the T Orange Line, roughly four miles northwest of downtown Boston. The Orange Line provides direct service to Back Bay, the Hynes Convention Center, Copley Place, the theatre district, the financial district, and northern and southern suburbs.
Destination	The Station Landing area at Medford's south boundary. There are several wind-down restaurant/bars here.

This route is shorter than our usual, but it is arguably the best route on the north side of Boston within the five-mile radius. It is excellent for anyone living or staying in the north of Somerville or south of Medford, and is also easily reached via the T subway.

Take the T Orange Line to Wellington Circle. Take the exit towards the west, and the pedestrian walkway to Station Landing, a comparatively new development with apartments, shops, and restaurants. Work your way west through Station Landing to the busy road called Fellsway or Route 28.

Cross Fellsway at the pedestrian crossing signal. Bear left to the paved trail and find the little footbridge heading off to the right. Follow the paved trail through the wildlife protection area to emerge by the edge of Mystic Valley Parkway at the entrance to Torbert Macdonald Park. This park honors a United States Congressman who served the district for 21 years. On entering Macdonald Park you find various trails

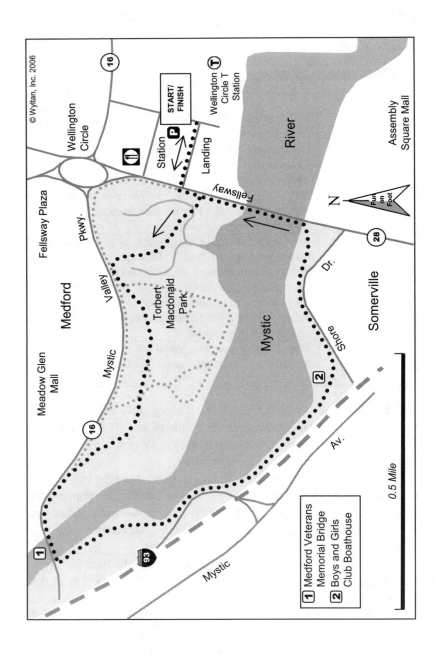

through a pleasant area, with traffic suitably distant from you. Our map and mileage assume the simplest straight path through the park, but the paths closer to the river are worth exploring. As you get to the western edge of the park, you are forced back towards Mystic Valley Parkway, and end up on its sidewalk to cross the Medford Veterans Memorial Bridge across the Mystic River.

Here you pick up a nice paved shared-use trail heading downstream along the south bank of the Mystic River. The only problem with this next stretch is the proximity of the Interstate 93 highway and its major traffic noise. Continue to the Boys and Girls Club boathouse, where you veer left away from the highway and pick up the sidewalk of Shore Drive, a quiet suburban street. After the bend to the right, you can veer to the left onto a dirt track through the river reserve, taking you to meet Fellsway at the Wellington Bridge. Cross the river on the sidewalk of that bridge and proceed to the Fellsway pedestrian crossing which takes you back to the Station Landing area.

At Station Landing there are several choices of places to eat or drink if you are so inclined. Nola and I like Not Your Average Joe's, but there are other choices including pizza, Mexican, and seafood.

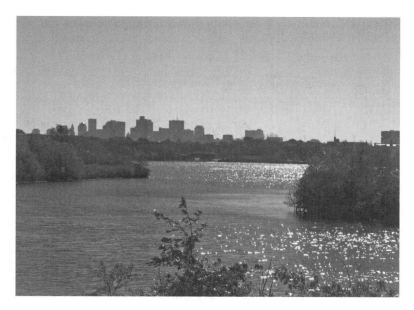

The Mystic River

Other Routes

Downtown Boston and its close surrounds present many opportunities for on-foot exercise. Stay away from the industrial areas (which are ugly) and use prudence in areas on the south side of Boston (including parts of Roxbury and Dorchester), which have bad reputations. Otherwise, you can comfortably exercise on-foot almost anywhere.

One popular route of note is the paved trail of a little over a mile around **Chestnut Hill Reservoir**, five miles south of west of downtown. You can get to the reservoir by the T Green Line to the Boston College or Cleveland Circle station. See our Finishing the Marathon route in Chapter 3 for a longer route that links up with this reservoir loop.

If you are seeking hill workouts, look to some up-down repeats of **Beacon Hill**, which is right downtown. Another good hill option is **Summit Avenue** in Brookline, off Beacon Street near Coolidge Corner. You can run there and back from downtown, making a nice seven-mile outing.

The completion of the "Big Dig" and redevelopment of the harborfront area have resulted in some new downtown on-foot trails. The **Rose Kennedy Greenway** is a series of parks that extend along the path of the old elevated Central Artery from Chinatown through the Wharf District and North End to North Station. In addition, the **Harborwalk** project has beautified the Boston Harbor shores from Fort Point Channel, around the city center and North End, to the mouth of the Charles River. The Harborwalk includes walking paths across the "new" Charles River Dam (not to be confused with the "old" dam, on which the Museum of Science is built), linking up with paths over the Charlestown Bridge and along the Charlestown side of the river. Recent developments there include **Paul Revere Park**, between the Charlestown Bridge and the non-pedestrian (Interstate-93) Zakim Bridge. Further upstream, there is **North Point Park**, accessible from the Museum of Science in Cambridge. While these developments are unlikely to excite the runner in training, they should certainly provide some nice places to stretch your legs when in the city.

At this point we conclude the chapter on routes within a five-mile radius of central Boston. The following chapter covers on-foot opportunities extending beyond that radius.

Enjoy Beantown!

3

Greater Boston: Inside Route 128

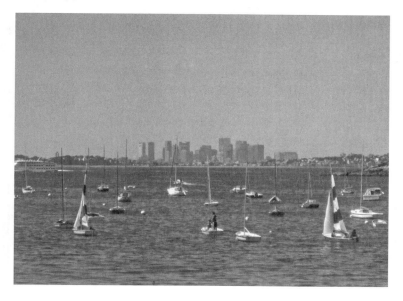

The chapter describes some excellent routes that extend beyond the five-mile radius covered in the previous chapter but are within Route 128, the ring road that to many people defines the logical boundary of Greater Boston. (This is not a precisely defined area, since Route 128 does not extend to the south shore, but we shall fudge our way around that.).

All routes can be reached easily via the T network, usually the subway, but in a couple of cases you need to use commuter rail. The commuter rail system is far-reaching and its quality is pretty good, but it is not necessarily very frequent. You should check the timetable at

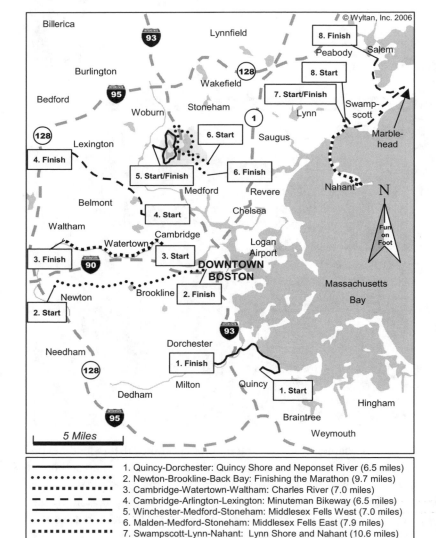

© Wyltan, Inc. 2006

1. Quincy-Dorchester: Quincy Shore and Neponset River (6.5 miles)
2. Newton-Brookline-Back Bay: Finishing the Marathon (9.7 miles)
3. Cambridge-Watertown-Waltham: Charles River (7.0 miles)
4. Cambridge-Arlington-Lexington: Minuteman Bikeway (6.5 miles)
5. Winchester-Medford-Stoneham: Middlesex Fells West (7.0 miles)
6. Malden-Medford-Stoneham: Middlesex Fells East (7.9 miles)
7. Swampscott-Lynn-Nahant: Lynn Shore and Nahant (10.6 miles)
8. Swampscott-Marblehead-Salem: The Path (7.9 miles)

Greater Boston Featured Routes (Beyond Five-Mile Radius)

www.mbta.com before embarking on an outing that depends on use of this form of public transit.

The routes in this chapter are ordered according to their position in a clockwise sweep around Boston from the south coast, through the western suburbs, ending at the north coast. If you want our personal recommendations as to top quality, be sure not to miss routes 2, 3, and 7.

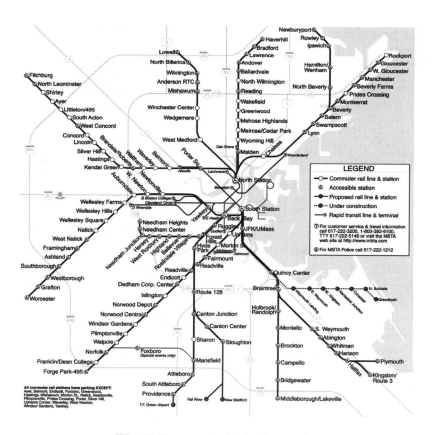

The T Commuter Rail Network[1]

Quincy-Dorchester: Quincy Shore and Neponset River

Distance	6.5 miles
Comfort	Roughly one mile is along regular street sidewalks. The rest is on dedicated pedestrian/bicycle trails either along the beachfront or off-street. Expect small numbers of other pedestrians or cyclists. Not suitable for inline skating in parts.
Attractions	A mix of excellent on-foot environments including paths through a natural park, along a marsh edge, along a 1.5-mile beachfront, and along a dedicated rail trail through the Neponset River Reserve.
Convenience	Start and end at stations on the T Red Line, roughly six miles southeast of downtown Boston. The Red Line provides direct service to the financial district, downtown shops, theatre district, Cambridge, and southeastern Boston suburbs.
Destination	The Lower Mills area on the Dorchester-Milton boundary. There are wind-down restaurants and bars here.

We included this route because its on-foot conditions are second to none and it takes you through such a variety of different environments. It starts in Quincy, birthplace of John Hancock, John Adams, Howard Johnson's, and Dunkin Donuts. You traverse Merrymount Park, the Quincy Shore, and Wollaston Beach. You then cross the Neponset River, and follow a dedicated rail-trail through the Neponset River Reserve.

Start at the T Red Line Wollaston station. Head north and east to the intersection of Hancock Street and Beale Street. Turn right into Hancock Street, pass Wollaston Avenue, and turn left into Merrymount Avenue. Follow Merrymount Avenue to its end, cross the street and go straight ahead to pick up the paved trail into Merrymount Park near the tennis courts.

Merrymount Park, with its wealth of natural forest, provides welcome escape from city and suburban life. Follow the paved trail to its end then take the gravel path to the north through the trees. It leads you to some sporting fields. Follow the road to the right to Merrymount Parkway, and turn left onto the parkway's sidewalk. Follow the sidewalk to the monument to John Adams and John Quincy Adams, father and son Presidents and two of this area's most famous citizens. Continue across the creek to Furnace Brook Parkway and turn left.

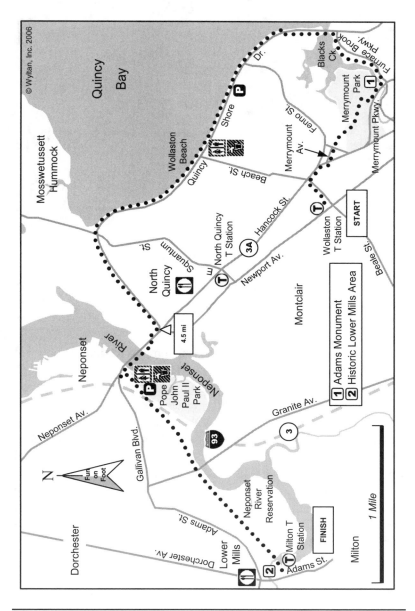

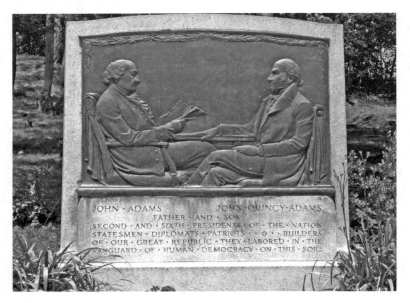

Memorial to John Adams and John Quincy Adams

Keep to the far left edge of the path along Furnace Brook Parkway. A dirt track peels off here and follows the edge of the marsh. If you like seeing marsh wildlife and getting away from all traffic, follow this track. Otherwise, use the street sidewalk.

After the track rejoins the street, you come to the intersection with Quincy Shore Drive. Turn left across the bridge and proceed to the picnic area and the pedestrian crossing light. Here you can safely cross Quincy Shore Drive to the beachfront sidewalk.

This is a very pleasant beach, with plenty of people on a nice day and views of the Boston skyline in the distance. There are restrooms at Elm Avenue, just before Beach Street. Keep following the beach roughly a mile and a half to its end at E Squantum Street.

Cross E Squantum Street and continue on Quincy Shore Drive. Where the road splits, keep to the right sidewalk and go down the ramp with the sign to the Quincy Business Area. Follow the ramp under the Neponset River road bridge. On the southern side of the bridge, climb the steps to the bridge walkway.

Cross the bridge. It is quite a pleasant crossing, with scenic views, although there is a lot of traffic close by. From the bridge you get to admire the new Pope John Paul II Park on the west side. At the end of the bridge, double back along the street to the park. It is a very pleasant, grassy park with plenty of foot trails, sporting fields, a water fountain, and seasonal portable toilets.

You can circumnavigate the park, but it does not lead anywhere. We recommend bearing right to pick up the paved rail-trail.

The Granite Rail Corporation (1826-70) was the first incorporated railway company in the United States. It was built to transport granite from the Quincy Quarries to Gulliver's Creek Wharf on the Neponset River for building the Bunker Hill Monument. Now its rail-bed serves us on-footers admirably.

Follow the rail-trail to Granite Street. To cross Granite Street safely you need to divert up the street and cross at the light. The trail from here on is very shady and pleasant, and is joined by the light-rail line.

Continue to the Milton T station. Here you can catch a light rail car, which is logically an extension of the T Red Line, connecting at the Ashmont T station.

If you want a wind-down break first, climb the steps from the T station and turn right into the Lower Mills area of Dorchester.

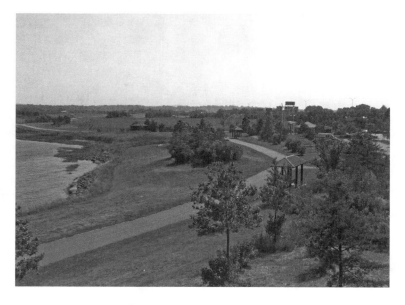

Pope John Paul II Park

Dorchester, established in 1630, was once the place containing the only powder-mill, paper-mill, and cracker, chocolate, and playing card factories in the nation. Lower Mills was the center of the milling activities into the mid-1900s. Today, plaques indicate the mill buildings that still stand.

There are a few acceptable eating and drinking joints around here. We enjoyed Donovan's Village Tavern and Restaurant in Dorchester Avenue, just north of Adams Street.

Be warned that parts of Dorchester have a somewhat shaky reputation today so, if you do not know the area, do not stray too far from here.

Newton-Brookline-Back Bay: Finishing the Marathon

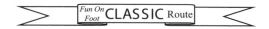

Distance	9.7 miles
Comfort	The entire route follows street sidewalks. The four miles along Commonwealth Avenue in Newton are very runner-friendly with pedestrian paths that are not close to busy traffic. You will find many other on-foot exercisers (but no crowds) here and around scenic Chestnut Hill Reservoir. The latter parts of the route are along busier streets, possibly reducing your running to walking in parts, but you will never feel lonely. There is little in the way of public restrooms, but usually a commercial establishment nearby in case of an emergency. Not suitable for inline skating.
Attractions	Experience the most crucial ten miles of the Boston Marathon route, including Heartbreak Hill. See pleasant scenery, especially on the part of the route through Newton. Pass several notable places and end in the heart of lively and historical Back Bay.
Convenience	Start at the T Green Line Woodland station in Newton, about a 35-minute ride from downtown or less from Back Bay. Finish in Copley Square in Back Bay, convenient to Back Bay hotels, the Hynes Convention Center, and T Green Line and Orange Line stations.
Destination	Copley Square and its many nearby food and beverage establishments. Attractions include Trinity Church, the Public Garden, Boston Common, and the start of the Freedom Trail.

The Boston Marathon, run every year since 1897, is the oldest annual marathon in the world and a prominent event on the nation's running calendar. It is also a very special event for all Bostonians, scheduled for running on a somewhat obscure Massachusetts holiday, Patriot's Day, the third Monday in April.

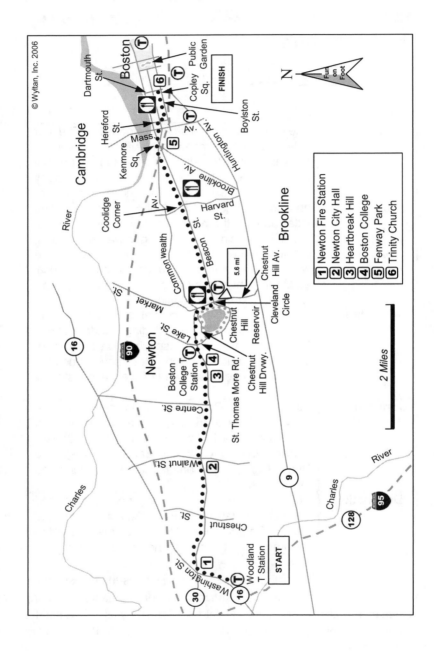

The length of the marathon, like all marathons, is 26 miles 385 yards. (This distance was set at the 1908 Olympic Games in London, being the distance from the king's desired starting point at Windsor Castle to the finish line in front of the royal box at the Olympic Stadium in London.) Whereas 26 miles is a bit far for the route criteria of this book, it turns out we can conveniently cast the last ten miles of the marathon course as a Fun-on-Foot route. This is the most exciting part for competitors and spectators alike. This route meets all our criteria well, with the special appeal that it gives you first-hand appreciation of exactly where the marathon runners are when you watch that race on TV every year. The last ten miles includes, of course, the infamous Heartbreak Hill, generally considered the toughest part of the course.

Start at Woodland T station on the Green Line D branch. You can catch this subway downtown at Government Center or Park station, or in Back Bay. The ride takes about 35 minutes from downtown.

Exiting the station, follow the sidewalk of Washington Street (Route 16) to the right or northward. Proceed to the intersection with Commonwealth Avenue (Route 30) and turn right past the fire station. This point, where the marathon route changes course near the 17.5-mile mark, is an important symbolic landmark for many runners. Unless there is a fire, expect to find the fire station's side door open and you can use the restroom and water fountain just inside.

While the Washington Street sidewalk is very noisy and not particularly pleasant, Commonwealth Avenue is a very friendly road for pedestrians and you get to follow it for the next four miles. Commonwealth Avenue here is wide and lightly trafficked. There is a grassy nature strip that pedestrians can use in parts and there is also a paved service road along the left-hand side that pedestrians can use, well away from any traffic. In January through April, expect to see many runners here, training for the forthcoming marathon.

At the 19-mile mark, near Newton City Hall, pass the statue of Johnny Kelley who competed in 61 Boston Marathons between 1928 and 1992, completing 58 of them and winning two.

The Boston Marathon is comparatively easy from a hill-climbing perspective since it starts roughly 500 feet above sea level and ends at sea level, presenting generally a slight descent throughout. The only major exception to this is the uphill stretch from the Johnny Kelley statue to the 20.5-mile mark, where the course peaks at roughly 250 feet above sea level. This arduous stretch is known as Heartbreak Hill.

Climb Heartbreak Hill. Since you are not in a race, you can do it at a pace that does not particularly stress you, but you can appreciate the burden placed on the marathon runner. The good news is that, after you reach the Hammond Street peak of the hill, it is downhill virtually all the way to the end of the marathon course.

After Heartbreak Hill, you come to the austere buildings of Boston College on your right. Immediately after Boston College is the intersection with Lake Street and Saint Thomas More Road, where the T Green Line starts following Commonwealth Avenue. At this point you have a choice as to how to negotiate the next mile. To accurately follow the marathon course, continue along Commonwealth Avenue, past the Evergreen Cemetery, and swing right into Chestnut Hill Avenue. Continue to the major intersection at Cleveland Circle and then go left into Beacon Street. This stretch, from Lake Street past the cemetery to Cleveland Circle, is known as the Haunted Mile. Considered by runners to be a jinxed stretch, it is where the legs and hopes of many marathoners have died.

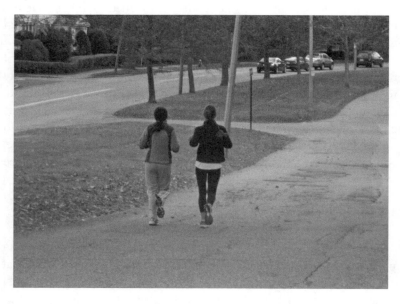

Runner-Friendly Commonwealth Avenue in Newton

VARIATION

There is a very pleasant diversion you can take here. Bypassing the Haunted Mile, you can negotiate the popular pedestrian path around Chestnut Hill Reservoir, a little over a mile in circumference. Go right into Saint Thomas More Road and follow it to the edge of the reservoir where you can join the encircling paved path. Go halfway around the reservoir in either direction. The clockwise direction is probably the more pleasant, in which case continue until after you have passed the rink and pool complex and then leave the reservoir on the path taking you to Beacon Street just west of Cleveland Circle. (If you go counterclockwise, exit on the same path, before reaching the rink and pool.) Cross Chestnut Hill Avenue at Cleveland Circle.

Proceed east now along the sidewalk of Beacon Street. This street is less friendly and more heavily trafficked than Commonwealth Avenue, but it is a wide street so still reasonable for pedestrians, including runners. From this point on, you have many opportunities to take a break or finish your outing, since there are various food and beverage establishments along the route and T Green Line stops in abundance.

Pass through the busy intersection of Coolidge Corner. After that, the environment becomes more pedestrian friendly, with lightly used sidewalks and traffic levels that are modest. Use either sidewalk but I recommend getting to the right-hand sidewalk before reaching Kenmore Square where you bear right into Commonwealth Avenue. Kenmore Square can be extremely busy pedestrian-wise, so be prepared to drop any plans for running at this point. If there happens to be a Red Sox game at nearby Fenway Park, then definitely forget it. Follow the right sidewalk of Commonwealth Avenue to Mass. Av. Cross Mass. Av. at the light and continue one block to Hereford Street. Turn right here then turn left into Boylston Street, finishing where the marathon finishes at Copley Square at the Dartmouth Street intersection.

VARIATION

If downtown Boston is your final destination, consider this variation. Since Boylston Street is usually crowded and not a good place to run, forget Hereford Street and continue on spacious Commonwealth Avenue to the Public Garden, Boston Common, and downtown.

The end of this route, Copley Square, is a short distance from many excellent Back Bay food and beverage establishments; attractions such as Trinity Church, the Public Garden, and the start of the Freedom Trail; plus T stations on the Green and Orange lines to take you wherever else you need to go. Pick your favorite destination before you even start the route, to help motivate you to finish it.

Cambridge-Watertown-Waltham: Charles River

Distance	7.0 miles
Comfort	Paved dedicated pedestrian/bicycle trail all the way, with a dirt runner's side trail in places. Some parts follow road edges, but there is generally plenty of greenery and shade. Expect to pass the occasional other pedestrian or cyclist but don't expect crowds, except possibly along the first stretch in Cambridge. Not suitable for inline skating in parts.
Attractions	A pleasant escape from the city hordes. There is considerable wildlife along the river and nice scenery. Waltham is known for the Waltham Watch Company, a key innovator in the Industrial Revolution.
Convenience	Start at the JFK Bridge in Cambridge, near the T Red Line Harvard station and Harvard hotels. Finish in Waltham Center, where you can catch frequent buses back to the T Red Line Central station in Cambridge, or (less frequent) Commuter Rail to Boston's North Station. From Central or North Station you can take the T direct to all hotels.
Destination	The attractive riverside city center of Waltham. There is at least one excellent wind-down pub/restaurant here, and the Charles River Museum of Industry (open limited hours).

If you liked the lower stretch of the Charles River described in Chapter 2, there is more enjoyment in store upstream from Harvard. There is a dedicated, paved trail extending upstream to Waltham, a historic city with a riverside city center. This route is different in character from our first route. It is much closer to the wilderness, giving better escape from the city environment for much of its length. It is also less used than the trail downstream from Harvard; so don't expect all the company you had there.

We have laid out this route as starting from the Larz Anderson Bridge (JFK Bridge) near Harvard. You can easily get there on the

T Red Line to Harvard or, if you wish, travel on foot 4.2 miles from downtown Boston, following our first route.

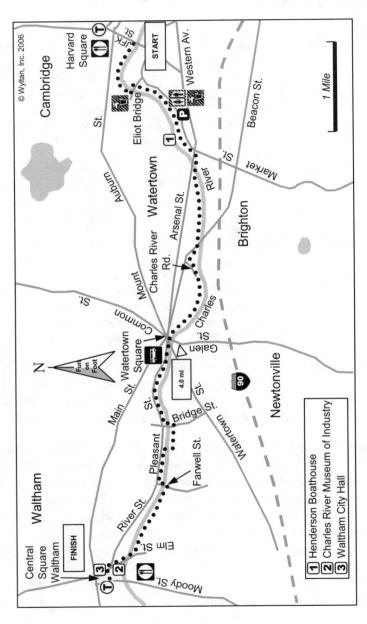

For the first four miles, from Harvard to Watertown Square, you can choose to follow either bank of the river. I shall recommend my preferred sides.

Start on the Cambridge side, following the river upstream to the next bridge, Eliot Bridge. This stretch is particularly pleasant on Sundays mid-spring to mid-fall, when Memorial Drive is closed to vehicles. Then cross Eliot Bridge on its left sidewalk, go down to the river trail, and use the pedestrian tunnel to cross under the road. Continue into and through a very pleasant part of the Charles River Reserve. Pass the canoe rentals, a playground with restrooms and water fountain, and the Northeastern University Henderson Boathouse. Continue to the Arsenal Street Bridge and cross the road here.

For the segment from Arsenal Street Bridge to Watertown Square, the northern side is the better, with a dirt pedestrian trail plus a shared paved trail for much of the way. Cross the river on the Arsenal Street Bridge and pick up the trail upstream.

Cross Beacon Street at the next bridge, then head north along the paved sidewalk trail. Charles River Road splits off to the left towards the riverbank. Follow the trail along it. You are soon presented with some pleasant options, such as an unpaved pedestrian trail close to the river for much of the way.

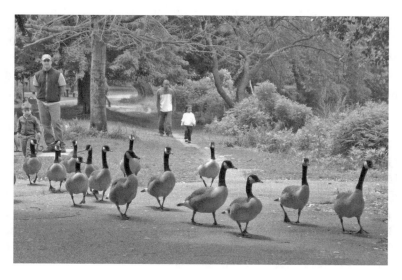

Wildife and People Sharing the Charles Trail

Continue to Galen Street at Watertown Square. Cross Galen Street. There are restaurants and fast food joints around Watertown Square and you can catch the Route 70/70A bus back to Cambridge if you do not want to go further upstream. However, we encourage you to push on, as the trail conditions improve now.

Continuing upstream from Watertown Square, you can start on either side of the river. The south side trail will lead you to a footbridge to the north side anyway, so you might as well start on the north side. The conditions from here up to Waltham are excellent for on-foot exercise. The trails follow the river—not the roads. There is plenty of greenery, shade, and wildlife. However, civilization is never far away—you catch glimpses of residences and local businesses through the trees.

You have to switch banks of the river a few times and—be warned—the signage is poor. Follow the trail to where it emerges on Bridge Street. Then cross the river to the south bank and follow the streets around until you find a little trailhead that takes you back to the river. Midway along this next stretch, a footbridge takes you back to the north bank. Follow the trail to where it next emerges on Farwell Street. Cross the river back to the south side here, and pick up the trail again along that bank.

After going under the old railway bridge, the trail delivers you out on Elm Street. The riverbank path stops here. Follow Elm Street to the right. It leads you into Waltham Central Square, where you can stroll, admire the City Hall, and find food and drink places nearby.

Waltham was first settled in 1634 and was officially incorporated in 1738. It is known as Watch City, because the American Waltham Watch Company, one of the pioneers of the Industrial Revolution, operated here from 1854 to 1957. It was the first company to make watches on an assembly line.

Bus and commuter rail stops are in Waltham Central Square. However, the commercial center of Waltham is a short distance away. Go to the west side of the square then turn left, following Moody Street back across the river. The riverbank here is nicely landscaped, with a little walking path to the west. There is also a path to the east that takes you to the Charles River Museum of Industry, in the 1814-vintage Boston Manufacturing Company textile mill. This building is on the National Register of Historic Places as America's first factory. Be warned it only opens on limited days though.

Possibly even more enticing are the shops and other establishments on Moody Street south of the river. If you feel like a really great place to wind-down for food and drinks, we can heartily recommend the Skellig Irish Pub. It has excellent food, including a brunch menu on Saturday and Sunday.

Backtrack to Waltham Central Square to catch public transit home. This route makes for a really great day's outing!

Cambridge-Arlington-Lexington: Minuteman Bikeway

Distance	6.5 miles
Comfort	Paved dedicated pedestrian/bicycle trail all the way, with comparatively few vehicle encounters. Expect many cyclists and some other pedestrians. Well suited to inline skating.
Attractions	A pleasant escape from vehicle traffic and a fascinating, historic destination.
Convenience	Start at the T Red Line Alewife station in Cambridge. Finish in the center of Lexington, where you can catch buses back to the Alewife station. (We recommend carrying a bus timetable.) The Red Line provides direct service to the financial district, downtown shops, theatre district, Cambridge, and southeastern Boston suburbs.
Destination	The center of historic Lexington, where the first fighting of the American Revolution occurred in 1775. There are numerous historic sites plus some good food and beverage establishments.

The Minuteman Bikeway is a paved rail-trail, which was completed in 1998. It starts at Cambridge's western extremity and extends for 10.5 miles through Arlington and historic Lexington, ending in Bedford. We feel that by far the most exciting destination is Lexington so, rather than describe the full trail, we feature the 6.5 miles from Cambridge to Lexington. You can then see the historic sights and catch a bus back to the start.

Take the T Red Line to Alewife station. Follow the exit sign towards Auto Drop Off Pick Up, then go straight ahead up the ramp or the stairs to Cambridgeside Place, the street that runs along the back of the station. Turn right along the sidewalk and proceed to the trailhead of the Minuteman Bikeway. The trail starts by taking an underpass under the Route 2 highway.

The bikeway is well marked so requires little commentary on my part. Follow it for 1.6 miles to Arlington Center where you need to negotiate some sidewalks to get across the intersection of Mass. Av. and Pleasant/Mystic Streets. Then continue the remainder of the route, with very few traffic encounters, to the center of Lexington, which you

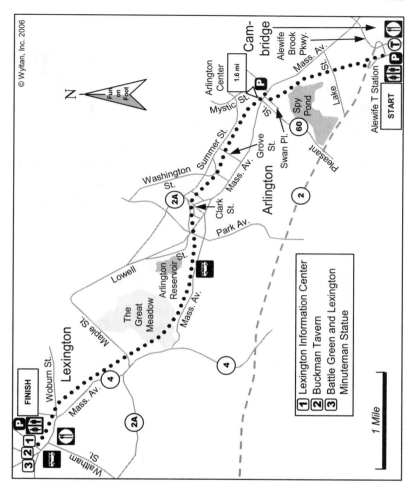

will recognize by its commercial activity and the restored rail station. Expect plenty of cyclists and a number of other on-footers on a nice day.

Exit the trail at Meriam Street, taking that street to the left to the Lexington Visitor Center, where there are restrooms and you can pick up a map to guide you through the local sightseeing. The 1710-vintage Buckman Tavern, which the minutemen frequented at the time of the 1775 Battle of Lexington and Concord, is nearby. Do not contemplate dropping in for a drink, though—this historical site is now operated as a museum by the Lexington Historical Society.

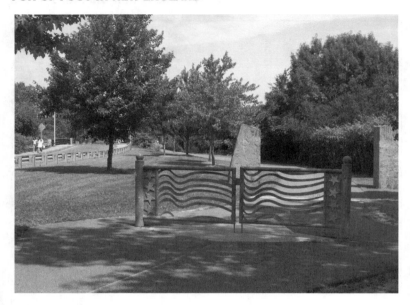

Cambridge Trailhead of the Minuteman Bikeway

Across the street is Lexington Battle Green with the famous statue of Captain Parker, known also as the Lexington Minuteman Statue (but do not confuse it with the Minuteman Statue in Concord). Also on Battle Green are several historical markers and the Revolutionary War Monument erected in 1799.

Lexington is not over-endowed with pub/restaurants, but there are a few choices. We can personally recommend Vinny T's of Boston, an Italian restaurant with a nice casual bar on Waltham Street just south of Mass. Av. Also Bertucci's on Mass. Av., with its pizza, salads, and beer and wine, is a good fallback. When done, catch the bus on the south side of Mass. Av. back to Alewife. We strongly suggest you get the bus schedule in advance, since the service is not all that frequent (half-hour to one-hour service, depending on the day of the week).

VARIATION

If you want to go further than the 6.5 miles of this route, you can continue on the Minuteman Bikeway to Bedford or, better still, switch to the historic Minute Man Battle Road to Concord. See our description in Chapter 5 of this fascinating on-foot experience.

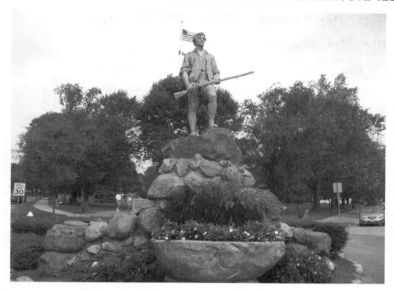

Captain Parker Statue, Lexington

Winchester-Medford-Stoneham: Middlesex Fells West

Distance	7.0 miles
Comfort	Up to 0.6 miles of street sidewalks then the remainder is unpaved pedestrian trails, mostly suitable for running but with some steep and stony spots reducing the pace to hiking. No vehicles and few bikes. Expect to pass other pedestrians, most often locals walking their dogs. Not suitable for inline skating.
Attractions	A complete escape into peaceful wilderness, with plenty of wildlife, history, and geological formations. Few people (but enough to keep you comfortable). Varied terrain, mostly thickly forested.
Convenience	If using public transit, start and end at the T Commuter Rail Winchester Center station, but the service is not very frequent. Alternatively there is a T bus service to Winthrop Street near Medford High School. If driving, there are a few parking lots, the most popular being Sheepfold, reached off Route 28 from Exit 33 of Interstate 93. Also see our next route for options combining the east and west sides of Middlesex Fells Reservation.
Destination	Winchester Center offers basic services. The appeal in this route is more in the execution of the route than in a compelling destination.

The 2,575-acre Middlesex Fells Reservation, in the northern suburbs of Greater Boston, is one of the most amazing natural resources you will encounter in any major U.S. city. It abounds with wildlife, history, geological points of interest and, most importantly, a wilderness escape for the region's lovers of the outdoors and of on-foot activities. It is managed by the Massachusetts Department of Conservation and Recreation (DCR) (formerly MDC), with the active support of the Friends of the Middlesex Fells organization.

However, the Middlesex Fells is on no tourist agenda. Rather, it is one of the best kept secrets of the locals, jealously treasured for dog-walking, wildlife-watching, community picnics, and escape from the urban world for anyone feeling the need for that.

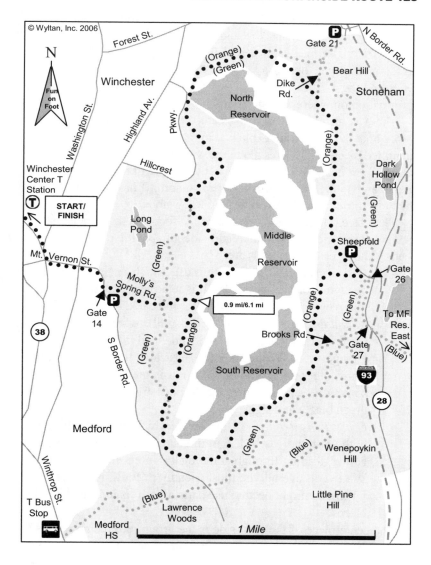

The Middlesex Fells is so large and diverse that we felt we had to divide it into two—the west side and the east side—for the purpose of suggesting Fun-on-Foot routes. The division is an obvious one—unfortunately the construction of Interstate 93 in the 1960s bisected the park in a devastating way. We cover the west side in this route description and the east side in the next. Some ways to build routes combining the two will also be suggested.

If you are seriously interested in exploring the Middlesex Fells, I recommend you obtain a copy of the definitive map produced by DCR and the Friends. See the www.funonfoot.com website for latest information on where to obtain one.

There is an extensive trail system, plus a network of fire roads, throughout the Fells, fully explained in that map. The various trails are identified by colored blazes along the way, but I must point out that not all trails are easy to follow because the visible blazes are sometimes sparse and sometimes confusing. I must admit I have become lost in the Fells more times than you want to know about.

Therefore, for this book, we decided to focus on three trails that are quite well marked, plus certain readily identifiable fire roads and public roads. The three on-foot trails are:

- *Reservoir Trail* (the Orange trail), which encircles the three reservoirs on the west side. It is relatively easy to follow and relatively friendly underfoot. It is indicated by orange blazes;
- *Mountain Bike Loop* (the Green trail), which also encircles the three reservoirs on the west side, and intertwines with the Orange trail. While intended basically for mountain bikes (most other trails prohibit bikes), it is quite well marked and sometimes a good choice for the pedestrian. It is indicated by green blazes and signs;
- *Cross Fells Trail* (the Blue trail), which connects the Fells, both west and east sides, from southwest corner to southeast corner, leading through some of the more interesting places. While not, overall, the most friendly of trails, there are times when you might need to use parts of it. It is indicated by blue blazes.

The centerpiece of the west side is the group of three reservoirs—North, Middle, and South—which are part of an active water supply system and are out of bounds. However, the encircling trails have much to offer.

For our nominal trail on the west side, we have laid out a 0.9-mile walk or jog from the T Commuter Rail station at Winchester Center into the Fells via Mount Vernon Street and the Molly's Spring fire road, followed by a loop around the 5.2-mile Orange trail. Then return to

Winchester center for a train home. While this is a fine on-foot outing, we recognize that, more so than with our average route, you may want to start somewhere else in the reservation or you may want to deviate onto other trails. Furthermore, the T service to Winchester is not very frequent and Winchester is not a very exciting place to wait for a train, especially if an alcoholic drink takes your fancy. We encourage you to use our map to help get you launched on whatever experience works for you here.

We shall leave the rest of the task of exploring the west side to you.

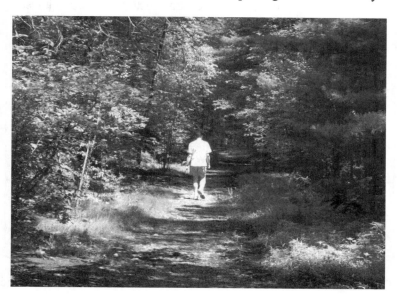

A Typical Fells West Trail

Malden-Medford-Stoneham: Middlesex Fells East

Distance	7.9 miles
Comfort	A mix of 4.3 miles on good, paved street sidewalks, 2.2 miles on mostly level, unpaved fire roads, and 1.4 miles on the Blue trail, which has some steep and stony sections not suitable for running. Expect some other pedestrians around, although the fire road and Blue trail sections can be quite isolated so you might feel more comfortable with a companion. Not suitable for inline skating.
Attractions	A mix of peaceful forested wilderness sections with plenty of wildlife and few people, and more populated but scenic sections around Spot Pond.
Convenience	Start and end at stations on the T Orange Line, which services Back Bay, Hynes Convention Center, Copley Place, the theatre district, the financial district, and southern suburbs. If driving, there are a few parking lots, the most popular being near the Stone Memorial Zoo.
Destination	Malden Square is a small city center with all the usual services, including a choice of restaurants and pubs. Have a wind-down snack or beverage and catch the T back to downtown Boston from the nearby Malden Center station.

The 2,575-acre Middlesex Fells Reservation was introduced in the preceding route description. This route is on the east side of that reservation.

The east side has some parts that are total wilderness, similar to the west side. However, the east side has many other activities. In particular, it is dominated by the large and scenic Spot Pond, with community boating, picnicking, a zoo, and some more conventional on-foot trails around parts of it.

Furthermore, the east side is acceptably close to Malden city center, which is blessed with frequent service on the T Orange Line and also some good wind-down food and beverage establishments. Therefore, we can much better craft a route here that meets all of our usual Fun-on-

Foot criteria. Our nominal route starts at the T Orange Line Oak Grove station, the closest subway station to the Middlesex Fells Reservation.

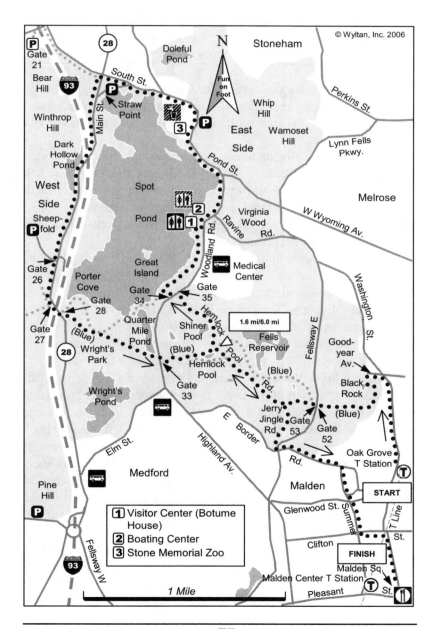

VARIATION
Rather than negotiating on-foot the southeast corner of the Middlesex Fells Reservation, which is one of the least friendly parts of this route, you can catch a bus to the Medical Center or other points around the reservation from Malden Center T Station. Check with the MBTA for route and schedule details.

Exit Oak Grove station towards the west, cross Washington Street, and turn right along the sidewalk heading north. You can almost immediately notice the start of the Fells, the area of rocky bluffs and trees to your left.

Continue up Washington Street, past a few small streets and around the bend to Goodyear Avenue. Follow this quiet cul-de-sac to the left. At its end, bear left up the trail and through the gate into the Fells trail system. Take the left-hand trail and pick up the blue blazes of the Cross Fells Trail, which leads you through Gate 52 to the north-south road, Fellsway E. Cross the road and enter Gate 53.

You then face some trail choices—the White trail heads off to the left, the Blue trail heads off to the right, but, if you prefer the easier and faster going, we recommend keeping to the fire road straight ahead and ignoring all side-trails. The yellow-blazed trail picks up the road for a short distance and then you come to a fire road junction. Turn right here following a very clear fire road. Pass the branch to the right leading to a gate to the reservoir. Take the left branch, Hemlock Pool Road.

You come to Hemlock Pool, which is the center of a major crossroads of the trails in this part of the reservation. We recommend continuing north on the major fire road, Hemlock Pool Road. (Say *au revoir* to the Blue trail for now.) You pass Shiner Pool on the left, a lovely pool, covered with gorgeous water lilies when we were last there. Ignore side roads and trails and you exit the forest at Gate 35 on Woodland Road. Cross the road and head 100 yards to the left, where you find Gate 34 re-entering the reservation. After a short distance you can see a road around the Spot Pond shore below you. Get down to that road and follow it towards the right.

This road follows the Spot Pond shore to Botume House, which houses the Middlesex Fells Visitor Center. If you do not already have the Middlesex Fells Reservation trail map, I suggest you drop in here and buy one. From here, take the paved sidewalk along Woodland

Road, heading north. Pass the Spot Pond Boating Center (open limited days May-to-September). The road merges into Pond Street. Go on to the Stone Memorial Zoo. Continue to the parking area at the northern end of Spot Pond, near Straw Point.

You need to leave the lake here and cross Main Street (Route 28). Follow the sidewalk on the west side of Main Street south and over Interstate 93. Continue past the reservation's Gate 26 (the paved vehicle entrance gate to the Sheepfold) and Gate 27, to the underpass under Interstate 93.

VARIATION

If you want something more adventurous than the Main Street (Route 28) sidewalk for this western leg of the route, you can enter the west side of the reservation and choose from various alternative trails in there. Cross Main Street at the pedestrian crossing at the South Street intersection. South Street becomes N Border Road. Follow its sidewalk to Fallon Drive. Go left, following the sidewalk under Interstate 93. Go left again before the industrial area and you come to Gate 21 of the reservation. Follow the main trail in, and at the first major branch:

(a) Take the branch to the right if you want to go around the west side of the reservoirs, following the Orange trail as described in our previous route description (End by taking Brooks Road to Gate 27). Alternatively:

(b) Follow Dike Road south if you want to simply take the Orange trail down the east side of the reservoirs and through the Sheepfold. Follow the Sheepfold sealed road almost to its exit (Gate 26), and then take the fire road south along the boundary of the reserve to Gate 27.

Gates 26 and 27 both lead to the sidewalk of Main Street, where you can pick up our main route description.

Follow the Main Street sidewalk under Interstate 93, crossing to the east side of Main Street. Enter the reservation at Gate 28. From here, we suggest taking the Blue trail, which is a little steep but quite well marked, to the south end of Quarter Mile Pond where you meet Woodland Road. Cross that road and re-enter the reservation via Gate 33. Follow the Blue trail (called Woodland Path here) to Hemlock Pool and the trail crossroads passed early in this route. Take Hemlock Pool Road southeast, backtracking part of your outbound route, to the intersection with Jerry Jingle Road. Take Jerry Jingle Road to the right, heading south to exit the reservation at the intersection of E Border Road and Fellsway E.

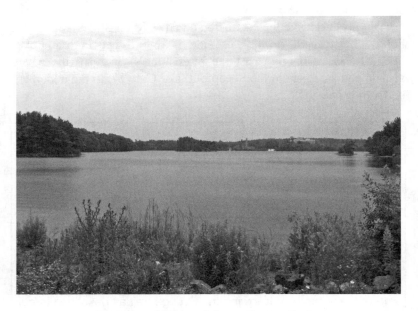

Spot Pond Viewed from Straw Point

VARIATION

If you want the fastest way back to the T, simply backtrack your outbound route to Oak Grove station. If you want to stop for some wind-down food or beverage first, follow our main description below to Malden Center. The latter option adds about half a mile.

Go to the left, cross Fellsway E, and follow quiet E Border Road. Turn right into Summer Street. Cross Glenwood Street and pick up Summer Street again, continuing south. Turn left into Clifton Street. Cross the rail tracks via the street overpass, and turn right into Washington Street. Continue to Pleasant Street, where the main retail area of Malden Center is to the left and the T station and City Hall are to the right. There are various food and beverage choices around here, but our favorite is Hugh O'Neill's Irish Pub & Restaurant at 45 Pleasant

Street. It is a great Irish Pub with good food, extended-hour weekend brunches, and nice décor.

When you have had enough, go back up Pleasant Street to the Malden Center Orange Line T station.

While this route is not without its challenges, we feel it represents an excellent opportunity for a different-to-the-usual Fun-on-Foot outing within the convenient range of Boston's T subway.

Swampscott-Lynn-Nahant: Lynn Shore and Nahant

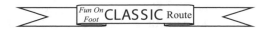

Distance	10.6 miles
Comfort	The first and last half-mile are along ordinary street sidewalks. Three miles out and three miles back are on a glorious paved coastal trail. There are three miles along the peaceful streets of Nahant and a half-mile pedestrian loop of a park at the tip of Nahant. Expect ample other pedestrians around in all parts. Mostly suitable for inline skating, except for some Nahant streets and the park loop.
Attractions	One of the most scenic routes anywhere, with views of Swampscott Bay on one side and the Boston skyline on the other. Plenty of sea air, and a good workout against the wind and some hills. A beautiful historic park at the tip. A very pleasant restaurant/bar area to wind-down.
Convenience	Start and finish at the T commuter rail Swampscott station, about 10 miles north of downtown Boston where you catch the train at North Station. The service runs daily but is not very frequent outside the main commute hours. If you drive, you can park on Lynn Shore Drive.
Destination	Some very pleasant seaside food and beverage establishments, plus small shops, on the Swampscott shore.

The north shore of Greater Boston has some scenery verging on breathtaking and, sometimes, we can craft a Fun on Foot route to take advantage of that. This particular route is our choice for the best north shore route within Route 128. We need to give credit for this route to Harry Greco, one of the most committed lifelong runners I know— Harry runs this route regularly and enthusiastically introduced it to me.

Start at the T commuter rail Swampscott station. Since the commuter rail is not all that frequent, I suggest you carry a timetable for the return trip. This route is, I must admit, mostly an out-and-back route, which is an attribute we try to avoid. However, as it is such a beautiful route, it still scores high marks with our selection criteria.

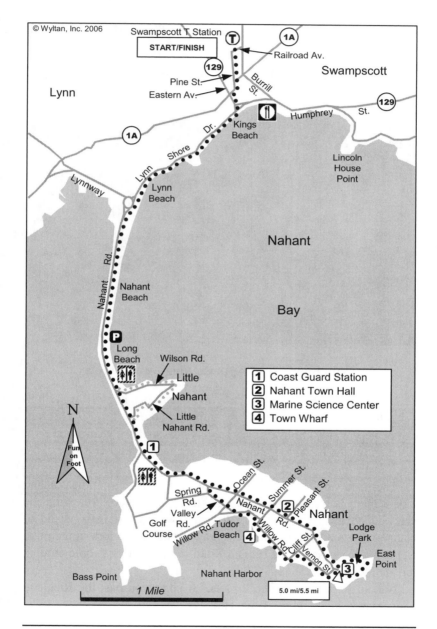

© Wyltan, Inc. 2006

Swampscott T Station

START/FINISH

T

1A

Railroad Av.

129

Swampscott

Pine St.

Eastern Av.

Burrill St.

Lynn

Humphrey St.

129

1A

Shore Dr.

Kings Beach

Lincoln House Point

Lynnway

Lynn Beach

Lynn

Nahant

Nahant Rd.

Nahant Beach

Bay

P

Long Beach

Wilson Rd.

Little Nahant

1	Coast Guard Station
2	Nahant Town Hall
3	Marine Science Center
4	Town Wharf

N

Little Nahant Rd.

Fun on Foot

1

Ocean St.

Summer St.

Pleasant St.

Spring Rd.

Valley Rd.

Nahant Rd.

2

Nahant

Golf Course

Willow Rd.

Tudor Beach

4

Willow Rd.

Cliff St.

Vernon St.

Lodge Park

East Point

Bass Point

Nahant Harbor

3

1 Mile

5.0 mi/5.5 mi

Exiting the T station, go right on Railway Avenue and at the end take Pine Street left one block to Route 1A. Turn right, pass the "Enter Lynn" sign, and then go left on Eastern Avenue to the shore. Pick up the paved coastal trail to the right, along Lynn Shore Drive. Expect many walkers and some runners around here.

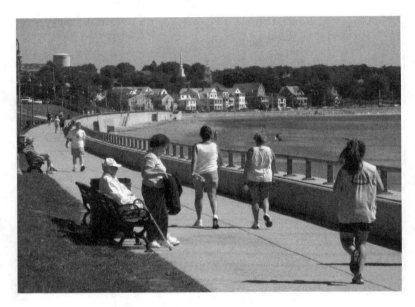

Lynn Shore Trail Approaching Swampscott

You come to the long causeway to Nahant heading off to the left. Take the paved pedestrian and bike trail along the causeway. This trail can be very windy. Snow is cleared in winter so it is a year-round trail. You can see the Boston skyline to the right and Swampscott Bay to the left.

The causeway takes you first to the small island of Little Nahant, where there is a restaurant and Dunkin Donuts. Keep following the sidewalk to the continuation of the causeway to the main island of Nahant. On reaching the main island, bear left at the fork in the road, following the sidewalk of Nahant Road. Expect other people around, mostly locals.

Nahant Road has its uphill parts. It takes you past the Richland convenience store and the Town Hall.

At the end of Nahant Road, five miles from the start of the route, you come to a parking lot at the Northeastern University Marine Science Center. There is a public right-of-way through the center's property into a fascinating place—Lodge Park, complete with a memorial to Henry Cabot Lodge. Follow the little foot trail and do a loop of the park. The scenery is spectacular, with a wide panoramic view of the ocean, including the Boston skyline in the distance. You negotiate WWII gun emplacements, largely undisturbed from their original state.

There are various ways to return to the causeway, including simply backtracking Nahant Road. We suggest continuing around the island via Vernon Street, then left on Cliff Street, then right into Willow Road. Follow the streets closest to the shore, around the wharf, to where Valley Road veers off to the right. Follow Valley Road up the hill and keep on it as it bears right back to Nahant Road. Now retrace your outbound route back to Little Nahant.

VARIATION

An optional diversion here is to circumnavigate Little Nahant. Take Little Nahant Road to the right and follow it as it weaves its way to the east tip. It leads to Wilson Road, which returns you to the causeway. The going is quite steep and challenging, so only do this if you want the workout. This diversion adds 0.8 miles to the whole route.

Continue backtracking over the main causeway to Lynn Shore and the point where you joined the coastal trail. You can go back to the Swampscott T or, if you want to wind down, continue around the shore a short distance to some excellent seaside restaurant/bars in Swampscott. We like the Red Rock Bistro and Bar. Without a doubt, this is a great place to sit down for a nice Sunday brunch after an on-foot excursion to Nahant.

Swampscott-Marblehead-Salem: The Path

Distance	7.9 miles
Comfort	A mix of 5.1 miles on good, paved street sidewalks and 2.8 miles on a pleasant, shady unpaved rail trail. Expect ample other pedestrians around but no crowds, except possibly in the town/city centers. Not suitable for inline skating.
Attractions	Some scenic ocean views plus some pleasant, shady inland trails. Optionally visit historic and scenic Marblehead Neck (add up to 4.8 miles) or Marblehead center (add 1.2 miles). Finish in lively and historic Salem center.
Convenience	Start and end at T commuter rail stations on the Newburyport/Rockport line (catch the train at Boston's North Station). The service runs daily but is not very frequent outside the main commute hours. Another option for returning from Salem to Boston in June-October is the high-speed Salem Ferry.
Destination	Lively and historic Salem center, famous for the witch trials of 1692. There are many things to see here, including the Peabody Essex Museum and the Salem Witch Museum. There are also several good restaurants and pubs if you want a food and beverage break while waiting for your return train or ferry.

Swampscott, Marblehead, and Salem are all very attractive places on the north shore of Greater Boston. We have put together an interesting on-foot route that links the three of them. This route makes use of a rail trail called the Nature Trail, or to locals simply "The Path," that touches all three communities.

Start at the T commuter rail Swampscott station. Exiting the station, go straight ahead on Burrill Street to the shore. Enjoy the sea air as you pass the restaurants that make Swampscott such a great Fun-on-Foot destination, as noted in our preceding route description.

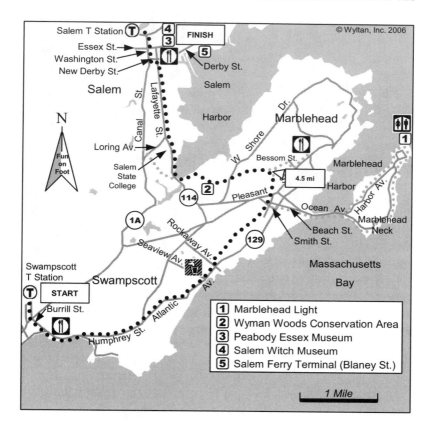

Continue along the main street, Humphrey Street. At the first fork, bear left following the sign for Route 129 East. While you need to use street sidewalks here, expect to have the company of a number of other pedestrians and cyclists.

Continue to the fork where Atlantic Avenue splits off from Humphrey Street. Bear right following Atlantic Avenue. There are elegant houses here, a good sidewalk, and a pleasant, mostly shady on-foot environment.

Pass the "Entering Marblehead" sign. There is a water fountain on the left at Seaview Avenue. Continue to Rockaway Avenue, where you turn left and quickly come to the rail trail. Take the rail trail to the right.

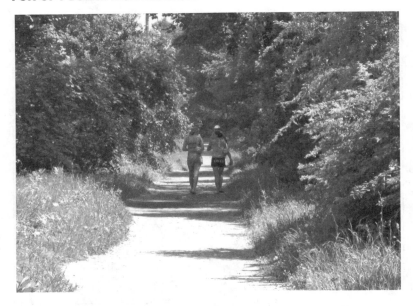

The Peaceful Nature Trail through Marblehead

It is a low-key rail trail—do not expect any signage or facilities. However, it has a wide gravel surface with plenty of greenery around and is shady in many parts. Expect other pedestrians on a nice day.

After passing the schools you come to an intersection with Smith Street. There is a convenience store on Smith Street to the left.

VARIATION

On reaching Smith Street, an optional diversion is to do a loop of Marblehead Neck, with its scenic views of Marblehead Harbor and its charming lighthouse. The full loop adds 4.8 miles to the basic route, but you can cut that shorter if you wish. Turn right onto Smith Street and then immediately do a dogleg left into Beach Street. Beach Street merges into Ocean Avenue, which crosses the causeway to Marblehead Neck. Enjoy the views of the historic harbor, established in 1629 and the place where ships were commissioned in 1775 to fight the British. At the fork, bear left into Harbor Avenue, which leads you past some impressive yacht clubs to the Marblehead Light at the tip of the neck (2.2 miles from the rail trail). Return to the causeway via the alternative road, Ocean Avenue, on the ocean side of the neck. Backtrack to rejoin the rail trail.

The rail trail leads you past a major power substation, where you need to bear hard left to pick up the trail to Salem.

VARIATION

From the power substation, if you are not in a hurry to get to Salem, you can easily visit Marblehead center, where there are shops and food and beverage establishments. This adds 1.2 miles to the route. Keep on the rail trail straight ahead under the road overpass. It leads to Bessom Street, which you can follow to the right to Pleasant Street. A couple of blocks to the left on Pleasant Street is Marblehead center.

The spur of the rail trail to Salem is like the first part of the rail trail, but with more wilderness and less suburbia. You pass through various conservation areas, and experience a nice escape from people and traffic.

The trail emerges at the bottom end of Salem Harbor on Lafayette Street (Route 114). From here, you have a choice of routes for the remaining two miles into Salem center. The simplest is to follow the sidewalk of Lafayette Street to the right, past Salem State College. Turn left into New Derby Street then right into Washington Street. An alternative is to cross Lafayette Street and pick up a short continuation of the rail trail northward. Cross Loring Avenue and proceed to Canal Street. Follow the sidewalk of Canal Street to where it feeds into Washington Street. Canal Street traverses a light industrial area so is not that beautiful, but it does have some services, such as fast food.

Follow Washington Street to Essex Street, the heart of lively Salem center, famous for the witch trials of 1692. There are many things to see here, including the Peabody Essex Museum and the Salem Witch Museum.

There are several good restaurants and bars in Salem, should you be ready for a food and beverage wind-down after your exercise. We have sampled and enjoyed O'Neill's Irish Pub on Washington Street, The Old Spot Irish Pub at 121 Essex Street, and the Salem Beer Works at 278 Derby Street.

To return to Boston, go north on Washington Street to the end, where you find the T commuter rail station. Check a timetable first, since the service is not very frequent. Another alternative from June to October is to take a fast ferry to Boston. The ferry leaves from the Blaney Street Wharf, off Derby Street.

Note also that there are plans to extend the rail trail inside Swampscott to Route 1A, not far from the Swampscott T station (the *Liberty Trail*). I have seen no progress on this yet but, if it happens, it will provide an interesting opportunity to shorten the route a little. Let us look forward to that some day.

Other Routes

Be sure to check Chapter 5 for other routes in Massachusetts, some within easy reach of Boston. Meanwhile, here are some other ideas regarding places that we consider to be loosely "inside Route 128."

The 7,000-acre **Blue Hills Reservation**, in the southern part of the region covered by this chapter, stretches from **Quincy** in the east almost to **Dedham** in the west. According to the DCR, it has over 125 miles of trails and hills up to 635 feet high.[2] It is a popular place for urban hiking and trail running.

Cohasset is roughly 16 miles southeast of downtown Boston, on the south shore. (Admittedly, Cohasset is not really within Route 128, since Route 128 ends long before the shore, but it is convenient to cover it here regardless.) Cohasset has some attractive scenery, and is reachable by commuter rail via the new Greenbush line.[3] The best running is the loop around Little Harbor, and you will find some pedestrians and cyclists around here on a nice day. Unfortunately, there are almost no trails or even sidewalks, so on-footers are forced to run along the edges of quite busy roads. Because of that, we are reluctant to recommend the routes here. About two miles southwest of Cohasset is **Wompatuck State Park**, which has 12 miles of paved multi-use trails and several hiking trails.[4]

Hingham is on the south shore, between Quincy and Cohasset. Near here is **World's End**, a very pleasant conservation reserve with such attractions as tree-lined carriage paths attributed to Olmsted.[5] However, the trails are not very long and the reserve is not convenient to a public transit system. At the time of writing, the only way to get to Hingham by public transit is by bus from Quincy Center or by Commuter Boat. While the latter sounds an interesting idea, I cannot recommend it because of the very shabby area in which the boat docks at the Hingham end. With the completion of the new Greenbush line, Hingham will be reachable by commuter rail.

The **Mystic Lakes** are a sequence of lakes along the Mystic River, upstream from the Mystic River Reserve, which we introduced in Chapter 2. The Mystic Lakes extend from **Arlington** and **Medford**

---

2   See: http://www.mass.gov/dcr/parks/metroboston/blue.htm
3   Scheduled for completion in 2007. Check with the MBTA for details.
4   See: http://www.mass.gov/dcr/parks/southeast/womp.htm
5   See: http://www.thetrustees.org

at their southern end into **Winchester** at their northern end. You can run around these lakes, although you will spend much time on street sidewalks. Note that these lakes are not far from the western side of the Middlesex Fells Reservation, so you can devise routes that involve both. Furthermore, a little northeast of Winchester Center, in the south of **Woburn**, there is a multi-use trail around **Horn Pond**, which can also be combined into the mix.

On the north shore, and within reach of the T Blue Line, you can find on-foot paths at **Revere Beach** and the coast north and south of there. This is a nice place for a run or walk if you are in the area.

Looking further north from **Salem**, we checked out running from **Beverly Farms** to **Manchester by the Sea**. This is a viable on-foot route, served by commuter rail stations at both ends. Manchester is also a very nice destination, with a beautiful beach and a good restaurant/bar. The main detraction of this route is that it mostly uses the sidewalk of moderately busy Route 127.

* * * *

Let us now look further out from Boston, considering first Cape Cod and the Islands, and then the rest of Massachusetts.

4

Cape Cod and the Islands

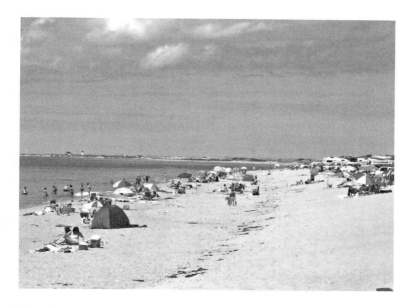

The number one vacation getaway place for Bostonians and other nearby New Englanders is "the Cape." Cape Cod is that absurdly large hook that hangs out the right-hand side of the map of Massachusetts. It is packed with beaches, campgrounds, holiday homes, marinas, day cruises, and other things that people seek for a summer weekend, week, or month break. South of Cape Cod are "the Islands." These are the two popular resorts of Martha's Vineyard and Nantucket, which are easily reached by ferry or air.

There are limitless on-foot exercise opportunities on the Cape and the Islands. In this book, we focus on a few key places that attract large numbers of visitors.

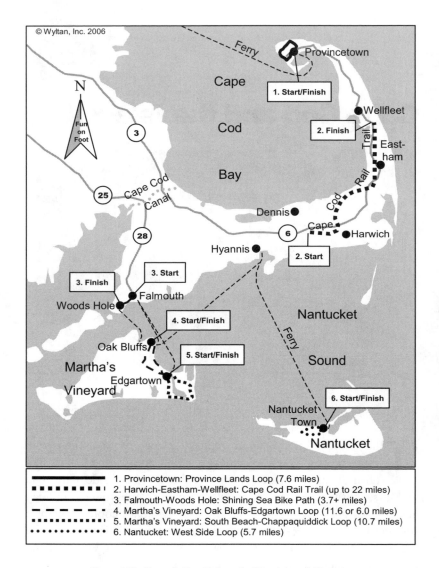

Cape Cod and the Islands Featured Routes

Provincetown: Province Lands Loop

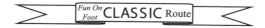

Distance	3.3 miles
Comfort	3.3 miles are along regular street sidewalks and the rest is on paved pedestrian/bicycle trails. Expect plenty of other pedestrians and cyclists. Not suitable for inline skating in parts.
Attractions	This route traverses a fascinatingly different environment, the sand dunes terrain of Province Lands, Cape Cod. Add to this the historic and tourist attractions of Provincetown and you have an enormously interesting place for on-foot exercise.
Convenience	Start and end in central Provincetown on the northern tip of Cape Cod. Provincetown is serviced by regular ferries from downtown Boston, making this an on-foot outing that you can easily build into a day trip from Boston.
Destination	Provincetown, with its many shops, bars, restaurants, and the historic Pilgrim Monument, which commemorates the first landing of the Pilgrims here in 1620.

Provincetown (known locally as P'town) is a uniquely interesting place. This is where the Pilgrims first landed in 1620, prior to relocating to Plymouth five weeks later. Today it is also well known for its large artistic community, its lesbian/gay population, and its summer tourist appeal.

While you can drive to P'town via the less-than-friendly Cape Cod road system, you can get there faster and much more conveniently from Boston by ferry. The ferry trip takes 1-½ hours, making for a nice day outing.

Apart from being a lively tourist town, P'town is an excellent place for on-foot exercise. It has a good paved bicycle/pedestrian trail system through varied terrain, including sand dunes. We document here one outstanding route.

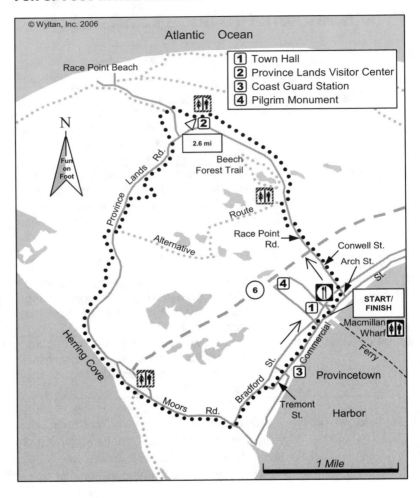

Start in Commercial Street near the ferry wharf in the center of town. Facing away from the water, Town Hall is one block away to the left. Take Commercial Street to the right and turn left into Arch Street. Continue up into Conwell Street. Cross the highway, Route 6, and enter Race Point Road. Follow the road edge a short way up to Seashore Park Drive, and then take the first street to the left where you come to a trailhead at the start of the paved bike trail system.

Go 0.2 miles to a car park and a branch in the trail. If you need a restroom, divert straight ahead a short distance. However, we recommend following the trail to the right, which is signposted to the Visitor Center.

> **VARIATION**
>
> You can take a one-mile excursion here to see one of the few remaining rich beech forests that were once predominant on this part of Cape Cod. Go through the car park to the trailhead for the Beech Forest Trail. Pick up a trail map and follow the loop around, then continue your main outing.
>
> Another variation here from our main featured route is to take the paved trail straight ahead following the sign to Herring Cove (marked Alternative Route on our map). This cuts 1.1 miles off our featured route but misses some of the more interesting environmental features.

Follow the paved trail 1.5 miles to the Province Lands Visitor Center. It is open April through November, and has restrooms plus maps and information on the flora and fauna in the fascinating sand-dune terrain around here. Then continue along the trail to the next trail junction, and take the left-hand trail towards Herring Cove.

> **VARIATION**
>
> After the Visitor Center, you can take a 1.6-mile excursion to Race Point Beach and back.

Continue on the paved trail that loosely follows Province Lands Road. Here you get to see some of the more interesting sand dune terrain, and its unique plant life. At 1.2 miles after leaving Race Point Road you come to another trail junction. Bear right and continue a further 1.1 miles to Herring Cove.

Herring Cove has a popular family beach (see photo at chapter head). Follow it down to the beach pavilion where there are seasonal restrooms and a kiosk. Go through the car park, bearing to the right and find a short paved bike trail here that leads you to Moors Road.

Follow the edge of Moors Road south. There is no sidewalk, but expect plenty of bicycles and some other pedestrians. You come to a road intersection with Bradford Street (Route 6A). Follow Bradford Street, which has a dedicated pedestrian lane on its right hand side (bikes on the left side). Take the first side-street to the right, then the next left into Tremont Street, which runs into Commercial Street a couple of blocks later. Commercial Street is P'town's main street and has some very attractive buildings. This street leads you back to the center of town.

There are many restaurants and bars in P'town, for you to wind-down while waiting for your ferry back to Boston. We particularly like the Governor Bradford Restaurant and Bar, which is a little more ordinary than some of the establishments around here. If you have time, also see the Pilgrim Monument and Museum, which commemorates the first landing of the Pilgrims in 1620. It is that big tower you cannot miss on the Provincetown skyline.

This is such an excellent route we have declared it a Fun-on-Foot Classic Route. Have a great day's outing here!

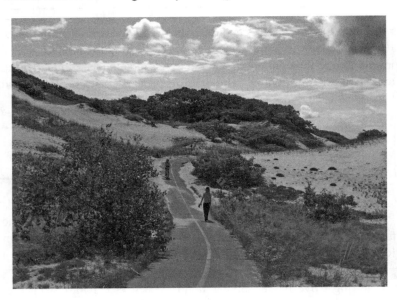

The Paved Trail through the Sand Dunes

Harwich-Eastham-Wellfleet: Cape Cod Rail Trail

Distance	Up to 22 miles
Comfort	A well maintained paved trail, with an unpaved shoulder for pedestrians and horse riding. You might encounter some reconstruction work in 2007-2008. Expect plenty of cyclists and some pedestrians. Generally suitable for inline skating.
Attractions	Passes through various Cape Cod towns and the Nickerson State Park. Passes through or close to several interesting environmental areas, including the National Seashore Salt Pond area.
Convenience	Start and finish at any of several access points in South Dennis, Harwich, Brewster, Orleans, Eastham, or South Wellfleet. The Cape Cod Regional Transit Authority's Flex bus service connects several of these access points, allowing you to craft many different routes of varying length with an on-foot outbound leg and return via bus (or vice versa).
Destination	Choose your favorite destination town, or other attraction such as the Salt Pond area.

The Cape Cod Rail Trail is a valuable asset for anyone living or staying in the towns it traverses. It is easily accessible from Harwich Center, Orleans, Brewster, Eastham, and, via a spur, Chatham. An excursion along this trail exposes the on-foot exerciser to most of the micro-ecologies of Cape Cod, including cranberry bogs, glacial kettle ponds, sand dunes, young growth forest, and salt marshes.

Because of the vast number of different options as to which part you may choose for your on-foot exercise, we have made no attempt to feature any particular part of the trail. Rather we leave it to you to craft your own Fun-on-Foot experience here.

To point out a few trail highlights, let us split the trail into three segments:

South Dennis to Brewster (8.4 miles): This stretch includes the branch trail giving access to Harwich Center, with such local attractions as the Harwich Historical Society Museum. At Long Pond Road, you

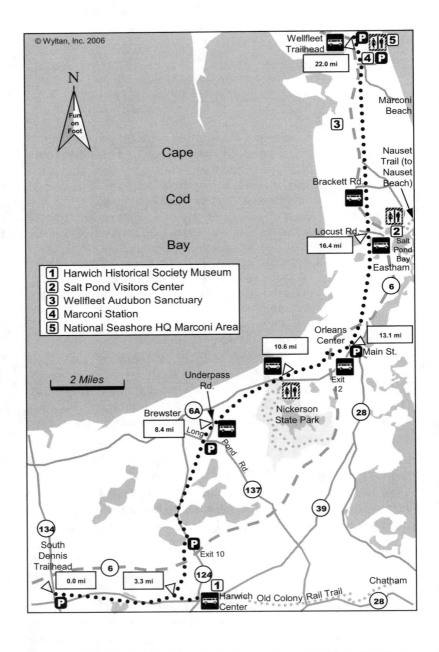

© Wyltan, Inc. 2006

N

Fun on Foot

Cape

Cod

Bay

Wellfleet Trailhead
22.0 mi

Marconi Beach

3

Nauset Trail (to Nauset Beach)

Brackett Rd.

Locust Rd.
16.4 mi

2
Salt Pond Bay
Eastham

6

1 Harwich Historical Society Museum
2 Salt Pond Visitors Center
3 Wellfleet Audubon Sanctuary
4 Marconi Station
5 National Seashore HQ Marconi Area

2 Miles

Orleans Center
13.1 mi
Main St.

10.6 mi

Exit 12

Underpass Rd.

Nickerson State Park

28

Brewster 6A
8.4 mi
Long Pond Rd.

137

39

134
South Dennis Trailhead

6

0.0 mi   3.3 mi

124

1
Harwich Center

Old Colony Rail Trail

Chatham

28

Exit 10

can divert left to the historic bayside town of Brewster, with beaches, marshlands, and ponds. Brewster also has many art galleries, craft shops, and antique shops, mostly along Route 6A.

VARIATION
From Harwich Center you can pick up the Old Colony Rail Trail, which connects to the coastal town of Chatham.

Brewster to Orleans (4.7 miles): This section of trail skirts 1,900-acre Nickerson State Park. Nickerson Park has over 20 miles of paved and single-track paths, mostly through wooded terrain.

VARIATION
Explore some of those Nickerson Park trails. The main trails do not connect directly with the rail trail but you can get to them at the park entrance.

Orleans to Wellfleet (8.9 miles): At Locust Road in Eastham you can divert to the right to the Salt Pond National Seashore area and its visitor center. Further north, if you like birds, you can divert to the Wellfleet Audubon Center on the left. Nearer Wellfleet, you can divert right to the National Seashore Headquarters and trails to Marconi Station and Marconi Beach. The Marconi area is where Italian inventor Marconi successfully completed the first transatlantic wireless communication between the United States and England in 1903.

VARIATION
From near the Salt Pond visitor center, take the multi-use Nauset Trail to Coast Guard Beach. You can then follow Ocean View Drive up the coast to the picturesque Nauset Beach Lighthouse. This variation is about three miles one-way. You can return to the Cape Cod Rail Trail via local roads or take the shuttle back to the visitor center.

The Cape Cod Regional Transit Authority's Flex bus service intersects the Cape Cod Rail Trail at several points, allowing you to plan an outing involving on-foot travel in one direction and bus travel the other. The main bus access points are marked with the bus symbol on the map. They include: Harwich Center, Underpass Road in Brewster, Nickerson State Park (seasonal), Main Street in Orleans, Locust Road near the Salt Pond Visitor Center in Eastham, Brackett Road in Eastham, and the Wellfleet Trailhead in South Wellfleet. Be sure to check the schedule and precise stop locations in advance at www.theflex.org.

There are various bike stores and food vendors along the trail.

Falmouth-Woods Hole: Shining Sea Bike Path

Distance	3.7+ miles
Comfort	A paved rail trail. Expect plenty of cyclists and pedestrians on this route. Suitable for inline skating.
Attractions	Beautiful scenery, including almost a mile along the beachfront. Woods Hole has some special attractions (see Destination below).
Convenience	Start at the Falmouth Bus Depot in Depot Avenue off Route 28. The Bus Depot is convenient to downtown Falmouth and is serviced by local transit and long-distance bus services from Boston and other points. If you are driving, there is free parking nearby. Finish at the Woods Hole Ferry Terminal, which is also serviced by local transit. Return to the start on-foot or by bus.
Destination	Woods Hole, with shops, museums, food and beverage establishments, and special attractions including the Woods Hole Oceanographic Institution and the Woods Hole Science Aquarium.

The town of Falmouth is in the extreme southwest corner of the Cape Cod peninsula. The Shining Sea Bike Path is named after the well-known line in *America the Beautiful*, written by Falmouth native Katharine Lee Bates. We cover the trail from downtown Falmouth to Woods Hole; the trail extends north into North Falmouth as well.

There is also a well-known road race run near here, the annual seven-mile Falmouth Road Race. Its course is from Woods Hole to Falmouth Heights, past Falmouth Inner Harbor, at the eastern end of Falmouth. You have the option of running part or all of this course in conjunction with the Shining Sea Bike Path.

We nominally start at the Falmouth Bus Terminal on Depot Avenue, off Route 28 (Main Street) at the western end of downtown Falmouth. The Cape Cod Regional Transit Authority's services, including the Blue Line and the seasonal WHOOSH Trolley, stop there. If you are driving, park in the free lot in Depot Avenue, at the skating rink in Skating Lane (add 0.3 mile), or in the parking lot on Locust Street (subtract 0.4 mile).

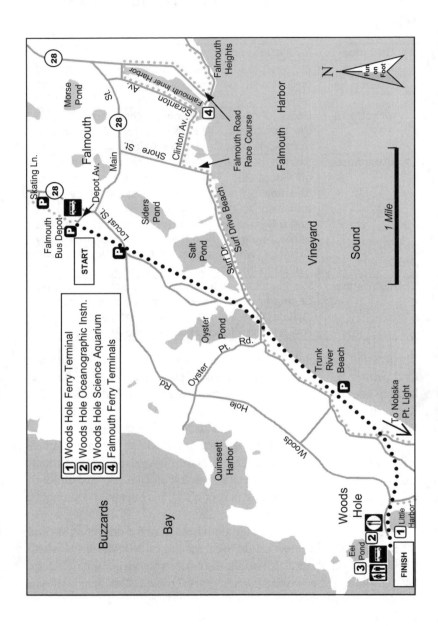

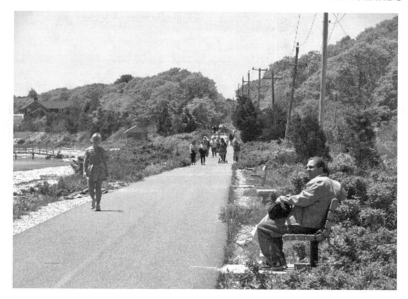

The Shining Sea Bike Path in Spring[1]

The Shining Sea Bike Path is very well marked, and you need no guidance from me to find your way to Woods Hole. Enjoy the variety of environments passed along the way, including ponds, forest, seashore, and bird sanctuary. The trail ends at the Woods Hole ferry terminal, where there are restrooms, food, and water.

Woods Hole is a popular summer retreat for Cape Cod locals and visitors. It has quaint shops, museums, galleries, and many food and beverage establishments, especially some very enjoyable waterfront eateries. You might want to sample the Captain Kidd Bar and Waterfront Dining Room at 77 Water Street; this is where the idea for the Falmouth Road Race was reputedly hatched in the early 1970s.

You can visit the Woods Hole Oceanographic Institution (WHOI) Exhibit Center and Gift Shop. WHOI is famous for the discovery of the *Titanic* in 1985. You can also visit the Woods Hole Science Aquarium. Established in 1885, it claims to be the first such institution in the country.

To get back to the start of this route, either backtrack on-foot or take a Cape Cod Regional Transit Authority bus, the WHOOSH Trolley, or

1   Photo by Kevin K. Lynch, courtesy the Falmouth Bikeways Committee.

the Steamship Authority's free bus to its Palmer Avenue parking lot near the Bus Depot.

VARIATION

You might be interested in using part or all of the route of the Falmouth Road Race. That route starts in Woods Hole, goes down around the Nobska Point Lighthouse, follows roads for a while, and then tracks the beach. It goes around the Falmouth Inner Harbor, ending in Falmouth Heights. Depending on where you are staying in Falmouth, this might give you an opportunity for varying your return from the Shining Sea Bike Path.

Martha's Vineyard: Oak Bluffs-Edgartown Loop

Distance	11.6 miles or 6.0 miles
Comfort	A paved pedestrian/bicycle trail all the way, usually along the side of a road. Expect to share the trail with plenty of cyclists and some other pedestrians. Generally suitable for inline skating.
Attractions	Pleasant scenery and excellent underfoot surface all the way. The inland leg is shady and peaceful, while the beach areas along the coastal leg are more scenic but more crowded.
Convenience	Oak Bluffs and Edgartown are easily reached by ferry or air services from the mainland. Ferries also service Vineyard Haven, which is about two miles from Oak Bluffs via street sidewalks. This route can be done as a circular loop starting and ending in either Oak Bluffs/Vineyard Haven or Edgartown. Alternatively, do a one-way trek from one town to the other, and use the Vineyard Transit Authority (VTA) bus for the other leg.
Destination	Both Oak Bluffs and Edgartown are quaint little towns with plenty of choices of wind-down pub/restaurants, shops, and galleries.

Martha's Vineyard is a charming island just five miles south of the Cape Cod shore. It is accessible by air or by ferry from Cape Cod, New Bedford (Massachusetts), or Quonset (Rhode Island).

In this route, we connect two of the island's main towns—Oak Bluffs and Edgartown. Both of these towns are serviced by frequent ferries from Cape Cod in spring, summer, and fall, and Oak Bluffs has some service year-round. The route can be easily extended at the Oak Bluffs end to Vineyard Haven, which has regular ferry service year-round.

There are two good on-foot routes between Oak Bluffs and Edgartown via designated off-road bike/pedestrian trails—one inland and one via the coast. Using both trails, we can construct a loop starting and finishing in either town. For description purposes, we have chosen to start and finish this loop in Oak Bluffs, which gives a total loop distance of 11.6 miles. We use the inland trail for the outbound leg and

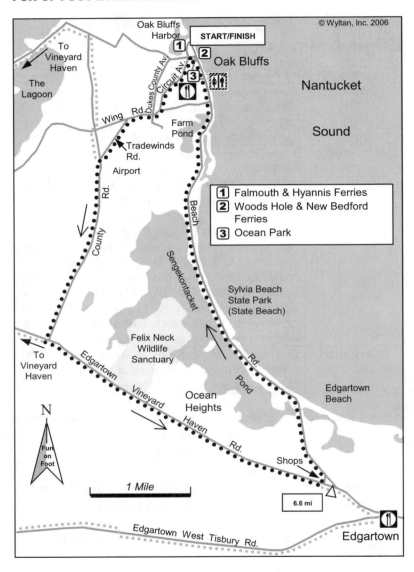

the coastal trail for the return. Another option for people preferring something shorter is to simply travel one leg of this loop on-foot then return via a bus service that runs in the busy seasons. For the latter option, we would recommend using the coastal trail, which is the more attractive, giving a one-way distance of 6.0 miles. We do not describe the latter option in detail, but its structure will be obvious from the map and our description of the full loop.

If you want to start or finish in Vineyard Haven instead of Oak Bluffs, add four miles for the loop or two miles for a one-way route.

Start in the center of Oak Bluffs near the ferry terminals. Follow the town's main street, Circuit Avenue, to its end and go right into Wing Road. You come to a quiet street angling off to the left called Tradewinds Road. Follow this street, which leads to a lovely paved trail to County Road. Cross County Road and pick up the paved multiuse trail to the left on the west side of that road. (Note that the northward trail to the right provides a good on-foot connection to Vineyard Haven, should you wish to start or finish there.)

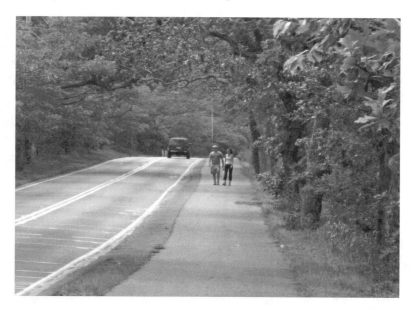

The Inland Trail Along County Road

Follow the trail to the intersection with Edgartown Vineyard Haven Road, one of the island's main through roads. In nice weather, expect the company of many cyclists and some on-footers.

Cross Edgartown Vineyard Haven Road and pick up the paved trail to the left, that is, eastward. (Note that the westward trail to the right is another way to get to Vineyard Haven.) It is a level and mostly shaded trail, well suited to running. The only problem is the noise of the vehicle traffic nearby. Pass the wildlife reserve on the north side of the road—there are trails through the reserve if you are interested.

At 6.6 miles from the center of Oak Bluffs, you come to the outskirts of Edgartown. There are some shops and fast food outlets here. If you want to go into the center of Edgartown, continue straight ahead roughly one mile.

To loop back to Oak Bluffs via the coast, go left through the shopping area and pick up the paved trail northward, along the west side of busy Beach Road.

After roughly a mile you come to the ocean shore. There is a gorgeous beach on the right, and a large tidal pond on the left, with the road and paved trail threading between them. Expect many people here in summer—maybe even the occasional ice cream vendor on a nice day.

Continue following the trail to Ocean Park, a very attractive Oak Bluffs park. After that park, go left on Lake Avenue and follow it two short blocks to Circuit Avenue.

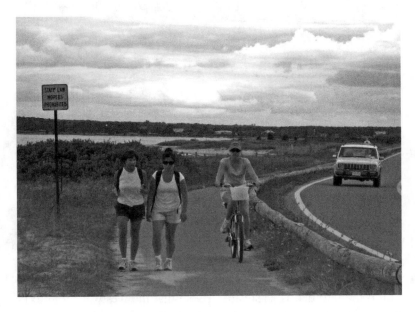

The Coastal Trail Along Beach Road

If you want a wind-down break after your on-foot outing, there are several pub/restaurants in Oak Bluffs, mostly in Circuit Avenue. We like both Seasons Eatery and Pub and The Island House Bar and Grill for this purpose. There is plenty to see in Oak Bluffs, including the nation's oldest working carousel (1876) and the "Methodist Campground" area of charming gingerbread houses.

If you finish your outing in Edgartown, see our next route description for what to do in that town.

VARIATION

The above route, starting from Vineyard Haven, going through Oak Bluffs, and then following the coastal trail to Edgartown forms the first part of the Martha's Vineyard 20-Miler Race. This race, run in February every year, is a popular training event for athletes preparing for the Boston Marathon, together with recreational runners. To complete the 20-Miler course, follow the Edgartown West Tisbury Road from Edgartown towards the west. Turn right into Airport Road. Turn right into Edgartown Vineyard Haven Road. Continue to County Road, where you turn left and follow our inland trail back to the Oak Bluffs School in Tradewinds Road. For more details, see: http://www.mvmultisport.com/20miler.

Martha's Vineyard: South Beach-Chappaquiddick Loop

Distance	10.7 miles
Comfort	The first 3.1 miles are on a paved pedestrian/ bicycle trail; the next 2.4 miles are on challenging terrain on either a beach or very sandy track; the final 5.2 miles follow quiet, low-trafficked roads. This route is no piece of cake, physically. Carry water. Expect ample other people around. Not suitable for inline skating.
Attractions	Pass through beautiful, sandy South Beach. Experience the fascinating environment of the Cape Poge Wildlife Refuge. Explore relatively secluded Chappaquiddick Island.
Convenience	Edgartown is easily reached by ferry or air services from the mainland. This route is a circular loop starting and ending in Edgartown.
Destination	Edgartown is a quaint little town with plenty of choices of wind-down pub/restaurants, shops, and galleries.

Edgartown, on the southeast corner of Martha's Vineyard, was incorporated in 1671. It was a major whaling port throughout the nineteenth century. Today it is a quaint town with tremendous appeal for the summer visitor.

Start in the center of Edgartown. Follow S Water Street to Katama Road. A paved multiuse trail starts here, following the east side of Katama Road. Take this trail to South Beach. This is a popular trail used by many cyclists and pedestrians.

VARIATION

If you are not inclined to complete this route after reaching South Beach, you can either retrace your steps to Edgartown on the paved trail or catch a bus back to town from here (in spring, summer, and fall).

At South Beach, head towards the left along either the sandy vehicle track or the beach. You pass a gatehouse, mainly focused on ensuring

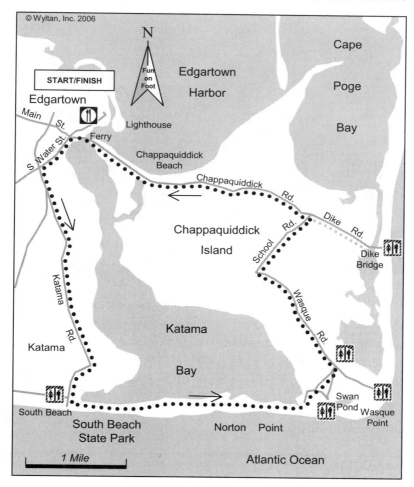

© Wyltan, Inc. 2006

N
Fun on Foot

START/FINISH

Edgartown

Edgartown Harbor

Cape

Poge

Bay

Main St.

Lighthouse

S. Water St.

Ferry

Chappaquiddick Beach

Chappaquiddick Rd.

Chappaquiddick Island

Dike Rd.

School Rd.

Dike Bridge

Katama

Katama Rd.

Wasque Rd.

Katama

Bay

Swan Pond

Wasque Point

South Beach

South Beach State Park

Norton Point

Atlantic Ocean

1 Mile

that any vehicles entering this very sandy terrain do so with deflated tires. However, we also found the gatehouse attendant extremely helpful with directions and advice.

Proceed along either the beach or the vehicle track for 2.4 miles. Be prepared to travel somewhat slower than your usual pace on this stretch, because of the sandy conditions. You then arrive at the Wasque Reservation and Wasque Beach. You are now on Chappaquiddick Island—or *Chappy*. If you follow the sign to the swimming beach you

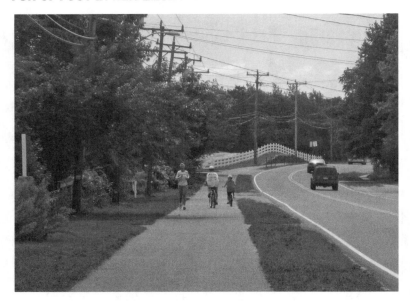

The Multi-use Trail Along Katama Road

come to seasonal restrooms and a hand pump for water. Follow the main access road past the gatehouse; where there is a soda machine should you need it. From here on, simply follow the paved roads. Follow Wasque Road to the intersection with School Road. Take School Road to the right, to the intersection with Chappaquiddick Road. Follow the paved road to the left.

VARIATION

If you want to see the famous Dike Bridge where Mary Jo Kopechne met her controversial death in 1969, take a diversion to the right at the prior intersection and go about a half-mile to the bridge.

Follow Chappaquiddick Road to the ferry and take the short ferry trip back to central Edgartown. The ferry runs continually every day and the fare for a foot passenger is very nominal. If you are ready for a well-earned snack or beverage, there are several suitable places here. We can particularly recommend Seafood Shanty, by Memorial Wharf on Dock Street, which has great food, great beverages, and a very hospitable management and staff.

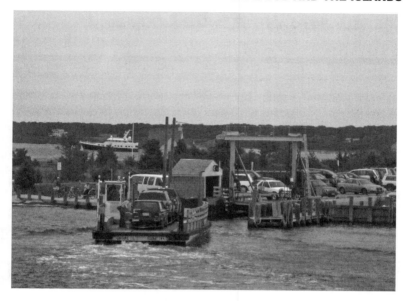

The Chappaquiddick Ferry About to Dock

Nantucket: West Side Loop

Distance	5.7 miles
Comfort	This route is mostly along street sidewalks and paved bike/pedestrian trails along the sides of roads, but there are short distances on road edges. Expect to pass other pedestrians and cyclists, generally relaxed and enormously enjoying themselves. Most but not all stretches are suitable for inline skating.
Attractions	Experience a great deal of what Nantucket has to offer, including quaint town streets, scenic views of the coast, beaches, and historic sites. Optionally visit the conservation areas of Sanford Farm, Tupancy Links, and Coffin Park.
Convenience	Nantucket Town is easily reached by ferry or air services from the mainland. This route is a circular loop starting and ending in Nantucket Town.
Destination	Nantucket Town is a charming town with plenty of choices of wind-down pub/restaurants, historic sites, shops, and the Whaling Museum.

Nantucket is an island steeped with history and charm. It was primarily a whaling center throughout the eighteenth century and through to the time of the Civil War. Since then it has become a place for escape from the pressures of the mainland, and a tourist destination in the summer months. The island can be reached by regular air services and by ferries from Hyannis on Cape Cod.

While there are many opportunities for on-foot exercise, we found one particularly compelling Fun-on-Foot route on Nantucket. This is a loop starting and finishing in the island's only significant population center, Nantucket Town.

Start this route in Main Street, in the heart of Nantucket Town. Be warned that Nantucket has very narrow streets; so be alert for vehicles at all times. Follow cobblestoned Main Street away from the harbor; enjoying the lovely buildings. Almost all Nantucket buildings conform to the same characteristic style, with roofs and walls of weathered wood shingles.

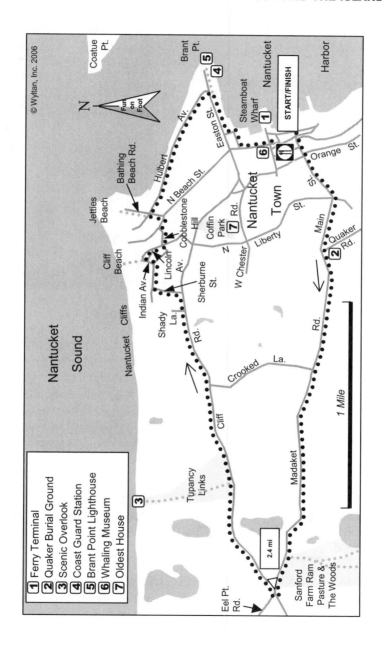

Nantucket
Sound

© Wytan, Inc. 2006

N

Fun on Foot

1 Ferry Terminal
2 Quaker Burial Ground
3 Scenic Overlook
4 Coast Guard Station
5 Brant Point Lighthouse
6 Whaling Museum
7 Oldest House

Coatue Pt.

Brant Pt.

5
4

Nantucket

Steamboat Wharf

1

START/FINISH

Harbor

Orange St.

6

Easton St.

Hulbert Av.

N Beach St.

Cobblestone Hill

Coffin Park **7**

Liberty

W Chester

Nantucket

Town

St.

Main St.

Quaker Rd.

2

Jetties Beach

Bathing Beach Rd.

Cliff Beach

Lincoln Av.

Sherburne St.

Indian Av.

Nantucket Cliffs

Shady La.

Rd.

Rd.

Crooked La.

Tupancy Links

3

Cliff

Madaket

1 Mile

2.4 mi

Eel Pt. Rd.

Sanford Farm Ram Pasture & The Woods

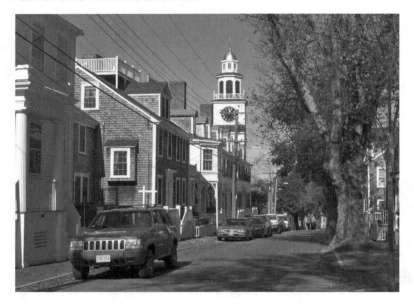

A Typical Nantucket Town Street

After the cobblestones finish, continue in the same general direction along Upper Main Street. After Quaker Road, a paved bike trail starts along the left side of Madaket Road. Pass on your left the Quaker Burial Ground, a cemetery since the 1700s. Continue along the bike trail, which is excellent for running, being level and sound underfoot. Pass the trailhead for the Sanford Farm Ram Pasture and The Woods, an area maintained by the Nantucket Conservation Foundation.

VARIATION

At this point you can add in a 1.7-mile loop of part of Sanford Farm to see some of its natural and historic features. This loop covers interpretive markers 1 through 13 on the guide maps available at the trailhead.

Shortly after Sanford Farm, the bike trail passes by the intersection of Cliff Road, Madaket Road and Eel Point Road. Follow the spur off the bike trail with the sign indicating Cliff Road. Go around to the right, crossing Madaket Road and then Eel Point Road, putting you on the bike trail following Cliff Road back towards the northeast.

Pass the trailhead for Tupancy Links, another Nantucket Conservation Foundation property.

VARIATION

You can follow the foot trails through Tupancy Links to an excellent overlook of Nantucket Sound above a 42-foot cliff, adding about a mile to your route.

Near the intersection with Crooked Lane, the bike trail ends and you need to follow the edge of Cliff Road for a little way. The edge is not wide but the traffic is usually light and fairly sedate. Pass Shady Lane on the left and then take the next left, Sherburne Street (there was no street sign when we were last there). Go to the T-junction at the end, where you bear right. Follow the first street to the left, Indian Avenue, which takes you to the loop area of Lincoln Avenue. There is a path here down to Cliff Beach, which you may wish to explore.

Follow Lincoln Avenue down towards town. You come to a most amazing street, called Cobblestone Hill, on the left. This street is right out of rural England—a narrow cobblestoned lane with high hedges on both sides. Follow this street to its end and go to the right into N Beach Street.

VARIATION

If you are more interested in the island's history and vegetation than the seashore, then instead of turning into Cobblestone Hill go straight ahead back to Cliff Road. Go left on Cliff Road. A short distance along on the right is the entrance to Coffin Park, a preservation area with pedestrian trails and a boardwalk through a wetlands area. At the southern end of Coffin Park is the Oldest House, designated by the Nantucket Historical Association. From here, follow W Chester Road back to town.

Take the first left into Bathing Beach Road, which leads to one of the best recreational beaches on the island, Jetties Beach. There are restrooms and a food kiosk here in the summer season.

Off Bathing Beach Road, take Hulbert Avenue eastward. It takes you almost to the Coast Guard Station. If you have a few minutes, go past the Coast Guard Station to scenic Brant Point and its lighthouse. Return to town via Easton Street and S Beach Street.

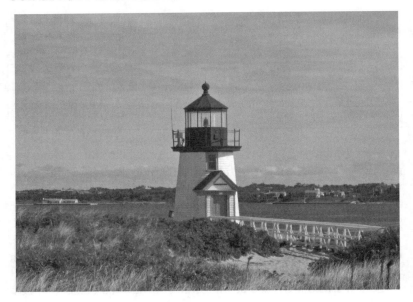

Brant Point Lighthouse

There are many good places in town for a wind-down snack or beverage after on-foot exercise. The places that we like best (and they continue operating outside the busy summer season) are the Rose and Crown and the Atlantic Café, both in S Water Street, and the Brotherhood of Thieves in Broad Street. There are many historic places to see afterwards, and be sure not to miss the Whaling Museum.

Other Routes

You can find many places to exercise on-foot on the Cape, generally along quiet local roads or, sometimes, on local off-road foot trails. Here are a few ideas.[2]

In **Barnstable** village, home to numerous sea captains' homes, you might try the loop Main Street to Commerce Road to Millway Road to Main Street.

The **Cape Cod Canal** has paved trails down each side, which are popular with runners, cyclists, and inline skaters. The scenery can be spectacular, running by the water and in the shadow of the high Sagamore and Bourne Bridges. Unfortunately, there is no way to do a nice loop, but there are various good out-and-back runs. The Cape Cod side can be easily reached from downtown **Sandwich**, which is on the rail line to Hyannis. The other side is convenient to downtown **Buzzards Bay**.

At **Chatham**, there are several excellent routes of various distances. For example, do a scenic loop from downtown as follows. Take Cedar Street to Battlefield Road to Champlain Road, and admire the views of Stage Harbor. Continue on Stage Harbor Road to Bridge Street, cross the drawbridge to Main Street near the Chatham Light, and return to the start point. Another place for a nice walk here, if you like beach walks, is Morris Island.

Hyannis is a major center on Cape Cod. An excellent loop here, starting from the west end of town, is as follows. Take Sea Street to Ocean Avenue to Hyannis Avenue to Washington Avenue to Irving Avenue. The Kennedy compound is on your left here. Continue to Scudder Avenue and back to the West End rotary.

On **Martha's Vineyard**, there are several trails in the **Manuel F. Correllus State Forest** in the middle of the island. You can get there from Edgartown via a trail along the Edgartown West Tisbury Road or from Vineyard Haven or Oak Bluffs via a trail heading south from the intersection of Barnes Road and Edgartown Vineyard Haven Road.

On the east side of **Nantucket** there is a nice paved bike trail loop from Nantucket Town, out along Milestone Road to 'Sconset, then north to Polpis and back along Polpis Road to town. It is a little over 15 miles, so out of our range. You can cut down the distance by taking

---

2   Several of these ideas are attributable to Geof Newton, who is working on his own, more detailed guide to Cape Cod running.

a south-north shortcut through the Middle Moors, which are interesting terrain in their own right. There are plenty of trails here but it is hard to pin down and recommend a particular route. Despite trying, we failed to find a route that we could confidently document for people trying to follow our directions.

* * * *

It is almost impossible to spend time on Cape Cod and the Islands without enjoying it. However, be sure to take what opportunities you can to get out on foot and maintain fitness while enjoying the other qualities of these places.

Now we move on to other parts of Massachusetts...

5

Other Massachusetts Routes

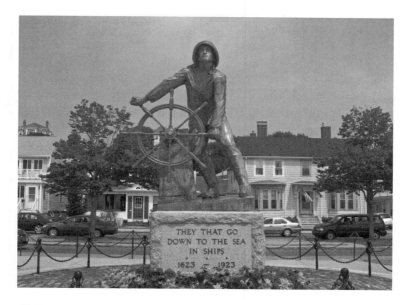

S ince Massachusetts—the Bay State—contains roughly half the entire population of New England, we afford that state much more coverage than any other state. We have four chapters covering parts of Massachusetts. The preceding chapters have covered Greater Boston and the Cape and the Islands. This chapter covers routes in other parts of the Bay State.

We describe two beautifully scenic routes on the north shore (in Rockport and Gloucester respectively), a gem of a route between Lexington and Concord (closer to Boston but just outside Route 128), and three routes in the more inland cities of Worcester and Springfield.

Of these routes, we have flagged routes 2 and 3 as Classic Routes—routes too good for you to miss!

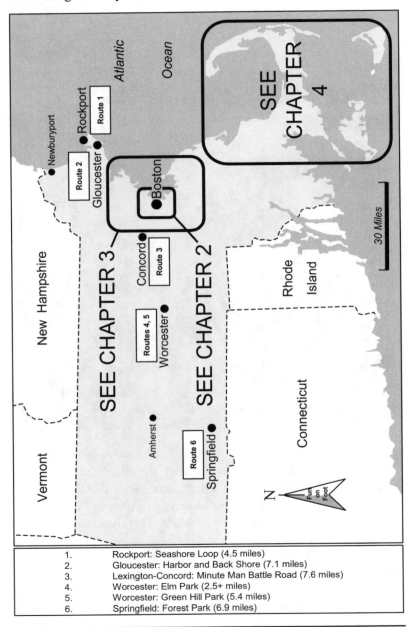

1.	Rockport: Seashore Loop (4.5 miles)
2.	Gloucester: Harbor and Back Shore (7.1 miles)
3.	Lexington-Concord: Minute Man Battle Road (7.6 miles)
4.	Worcester: Elm Park (2.5+ miles)
5.	Worcester: Green Hill Park (5.4 miles)
6.	Springfield: Forest Park (6.9 miles)

Rockport: Seashore Loop

Distance	4.5 miles
Comfort	The route is along street sidewalks, except for 0.4 miles on narrow, natural footpaths. Expect plenty of other people around. Parts of the route can be crowded on a busy summer weekend or holiday. Not suitable for inline skating.
Attractions	A picturesque seaside town and some beautiful scenery involving the ocean, beaches, and rocky headlands.
Convenience	Start and end at the T commuter rail Rockport station. You can catch the train to here from Boston's North Station.
Destination	The quaint town center of Rockport, with plenty of shops and restaurants.

Rockport, which hugs the Atlantic coastline around the northeast corner of Cape Ann, is as picturesque as towns get. This route weaves through the town and takes you past some of the most spectacular ocean views, making use of some little-known footpaths.

Start at the T commuter rail station on Railroad Avenue. Follow Railroad Avenue to the left. It becomes Granite Street. Follow the sidewalk, along a pleasant tree-lined road with light traffic, to the seashore at Beach Street.

Turn right and pick up the paved seaside trail along Beach Street. On your left is Back Beach, with a lovely view of the town. Continue to Front Beach, where Beach Street runs into Main Street. Continue past Bearskin Neck, with its shops and harbor views that you may want to check out later. Proceed around the harbor, bearing left into Atlantic Avenue.

Follow Atlantic Avenue to where it swings right, and find the entrance to the "Public Footpath" here. Take the footpath to where it emerges on The Headlands. The scenery here, atop an exposed rocky outcrop, is nothing short of breathtaking. Cross The Headlands, without going down the cliffs, and find a new trail starting on the other side. Note that you do not want to go away from the sea towards the houses, since that direction leads to private property. The trail takes you to the west end of Old Garden Road.

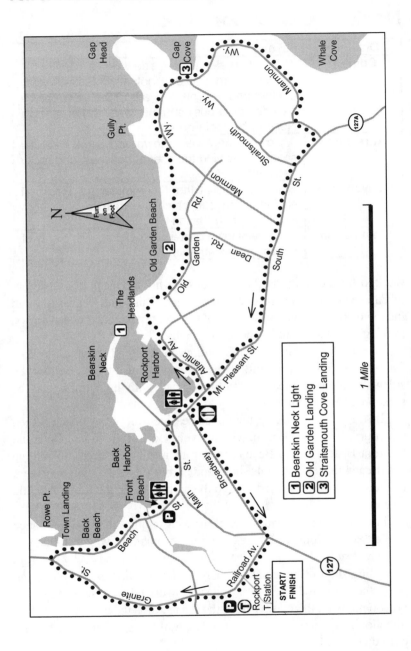

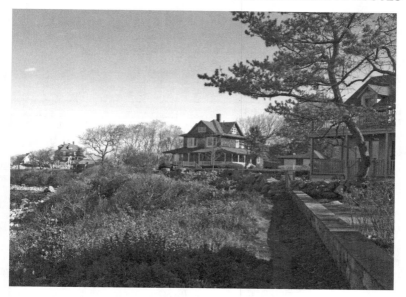

The Footpath Above Old Garden Beach

Follow Old Garden Road eastward to its intersection with Dean Road, where there is an access path on the left to yet another footpath. This quaint little path takes you along the cliff above scenic Old Garden Beach. Follow the path to its end, where it emerges on Marmion Way.

Turn left and follow Marmion Way past Gully Point to Straitsmouth Cove Landing where, according to the sign, fishermen started fishing in the 1600s.

Continue following Marmion Way past attractive houses to its end at South Street (Route 127A). Turn right on South Street and follow its sidewalk back to the town center. To get back to the T station, follow either Broadway or Main Street to Railroad Avenue.

In addition to plenty of shops, there are several cafes and restaurants in the town center. There are no bars. Rockport was a dry town since before the Civil War, and it was only in 2005 that restaurants started serving alcohol with food.

Gloucester: Harbor and Back Shore

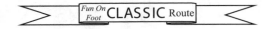

Distance	7.1 miles
Comfort	The entire route is along street sidewalks, the quality of which varies from narrow and bumpy to wide and smooth. However, nearby traffic is low volume and kept slow by tight speed limits. Expect plenty of other pedestrians. Not generally suitable for inline skating.
Attractions	This is an extremely interesting and scenic route. You get to see all aspects of the fishing industry for which Gloucester is so famous. Pass the Fishermen's Memorial, the Crow's Nest Bar used to film *The Perfect Storm*, and the State Fish Pier. Also pass by the Rocky Neck art colony and some popular, sandy beaches, and experience an ocean-side trail above the cliffs with outstanding scenery.
Convenience	Start and end in central Gloucester. Gloucester can be reached by the T commuter rail system from Boston's North Station. If driving, simply follow Route 128 to its northern end.
Destination	Gloucester, with its shops, bars, restaurants, and fishing industry monuments and memorabilia.

Gloucester is the oldest working fishing port in the United States, first settled in 1623. It is also the location of the October 1991 "storm of the century" featured in Sebastian Junger's book *The Perfect Storm* and the Warner Bros. movie of the same name. There is just so much fishing industry history here, plus such lovely scenery, you cannot fail to enjoy having Fun on Foot in Gloucester. The route we have chosen, we believe, captures the best aspects of everything this city has to offer.

We nominally start and finish the route at the Fishermen's Memorial, Gloucester's most famous landmark. The "Man at the Wheel" statue, sculpted by Leonard Craske, commemorates "They that go down to the sea in ships." (See photo at head of chapter.)

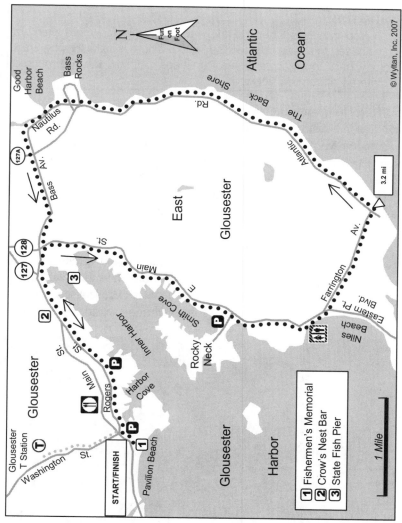

If you take the commuter rail to Gloucester station, go down Washington Street to pick up our route (add 0.2 miles on outbound and return if you do this). If you are driving, park near the memorial.

Follow the sidewalk of Route 127 eastward through the city center. Pass the Crow's Nest Bar, made famous in *The Perfect Storm*. Continue around the harbor and above the State Fish Pier. At the traffic signal, follow the sign to East Gloucester—this is E Main Street. Continue along the sidewalk to Rocky Neck Avenue on the right.

> **VARIATION**
> You can divert here to explore Rocky Neck, where painters have based themselves since the 1890s. There is still a thriving artist colony here today, plus several galleries. Follow the red-marked Painters Path on the sidewalk.

Keep following the sidewalk to the start of Niles Beach. There are seasonal restrooms here. At the security gates, head to the left up Farrington Avenue. (If you go through the gates and around the shore you get to Eastern Point with a spectacular view, although you need to use what is marked as a private road.) There is no sidewalk on Farrington but an adequate verge for walking or running. The traffic is light and, with a 25-mph posted speed limit, vehicles move sedately. Expect other pedestrians on this route and the occasional bike.

At the 3.2-mile mark you meet Atlantic Road. Follow it to the left. There is a good sidewalk now. The first part is shady, until the road starts following the oceanfront. This part is known as the Back Shore, and is very popular with local joggers. There are excellent scenic views of the ocean, the rocks below, and some charming seaside dwellings.

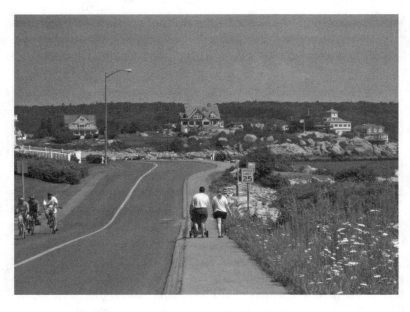

Scenic Pedestrian-Friendly Atlantic Road

At the 3.9-mile point, you come to an intersection where vehicles are forced to turn left inland. We recommend going straight ahead into the one-way southbound street, Nautilus Road. This takes you past the Bass Rocks area with its quaint seaside residences. You then pass the overlook of the beautiful, long, and sandy Good Harbor Beach.

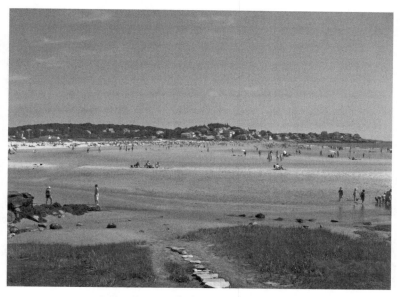

Sandy and Popular Good Harbor Beach

Follow Nautilus Road around to a major road intersection, where you go straight ahead into Bass Avenue. Pass a group of shops on the right. You then come to another major intersection with a traffic signal, where Route 128 starts. Continue straight ahead into Main Street, now retracing the steps of the first part of the route.

Follow Main Street or Rogers Street through the city center back to the Fishermen's Memorial, or turn right into Washington Street if you want the T station.

If you feel like a food or beverage break, there are several restaurants and a few taverns in the city center. I have sampled the Pilot House on Rogers Street and the Blackburn Tavern on Main Street at Washington Street. Both are reasonably priced restaurant/bars with quite good quality food, including plenty of seafood choices. The Blackburn Tavern has a jazz brunch on Sundays.

Lexington-Concord: Minute Man Battle Road

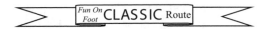

Distance	7.6 miles
Comfort	The first 1.5 and last 1.8 miles are on street sidewalks and the rest is on a well-marked multi-use trail shared by pedestrians and bikes. Expect plenty of other pedestrians around, including both joggers and more sedate history buffs. While inline skating is possible, the surface is very rough in parts.
Attractions	Pass through the fascinating Minute Man National Historical Park with its many informative markers and restorations, while enjoying the peaceful, shaded trail. Also pass by many other historical sites close to Concord and Lexington, including The Wayside, the home of three famous 19th century literary families.
Convenience	Lexington is reachable by T bus service from the T Red Line Alewife station, and Concord is reachable by T commuter rail from Boston's North Station. Since services are not very frequent, you should check timetables in advance.
Destination	Both Concord and Lexington are very interesting destinations, with many historical sites, museums, restaurants, and some bars.

The fighting of the American Revolution began on April 19, 1775, with the firing of shots at the North Bridge in Concord, Massachusetts, followed by a series of skirmishes along the road of British retreat from Concord through Lexington to Boston. A great deal of the history and character of that place at that time has been captured in the Minute Man National Historical Park, embracing a major part of that road between Concord and Lexington.

The best way to experience that scene is unquestionably on-foot along the 4.3-mile Minute Man Battle Road Trail. To help you do this, we have constructed a 7.6-mile Fun on Foot route between the centers of Lexington and Concord, both of which can be reached by public transit via the T network.

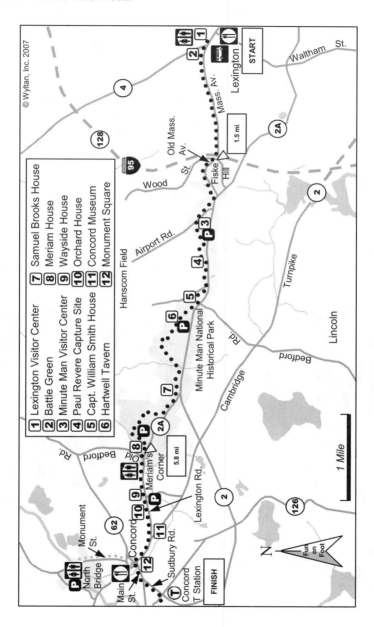

You can do this route in either direction. Despite going against the direction of the British retreat, we have chosen to favor the direction Lexington-to-Concord. Because Concord is such a charming and fascinating town, you may appreciate the opportunity to spend a significant time here after completing your on-foot route. If you want to go the opposite way, you should find that straightforward given the information we include here.

You can get to Lexington by bus from the T Red Line Alewife station at Cambridge's western edge. Alternatively, if you feel like an exhilarating 14-mile training run, take the Minuteman Bikeway from Alewife to Lexington (as described in Chapter 3) and then tack on this route. On arrival in Lexington, you can pick up a map of the Battle Road Trail at the Visitor Center on Mass. Av. near Battle Green.

Cross the street to the Captain Parker Statue, and then proceed westward on the sidewalk of Mass. Av., with Battle Green on your right. You climb a rise and then go downhill to where you cross Interstate 95. On the other side of the highway, turn right then immediately left into Old Mass. Av. Here, 1.5 miles from the start, you find the eastern end of the Battle Road Trail.

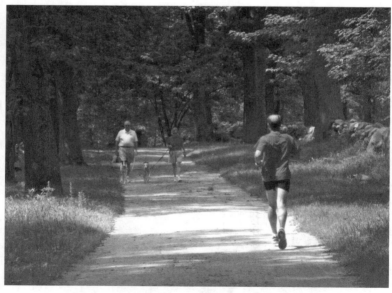

Sharing the Battle Road Trail

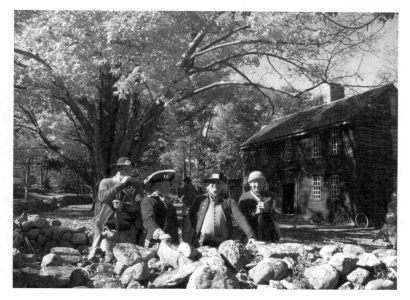

Redcoats at the Hartwell Tavern[1]

The Battle Road Trail is one of the most fascinating and enjoyable on-foot trails we have encountered anywhere. Not only does it have its outstanding historic attractions and a unique atmosphere, but it is also a particularly pleasant environment for running, jogging, or walking. You will find just as many people focused on exercise around here as you will find history students.

Follow the well-marked trail and read the historical markers that interest you. You pass the Minute Man Visitor Center, a plaque marking where Paul Revere's midnight ride came to an end, several restored buildings of the period, and several other points of historical interest. Do not be surprised to find helpful people in period costume at various places, such as the 1733-vintage Hartwell Tavern. Continue to where the trail ends at Meriam's corner, where the shots exchanged between colonial militia and British troops began the fighting along the Battle Road. There are restrooms and water available at Meriam's corner.

Cross Old Bedford Road and continue west along the sidewalk of Lexington Road. It is a very pleasant 1.3-mile run, jog, or walk to Concord center. You pass some very impressive houses, several

1   Photo courtesy National Parks Service.

of historical significance, and the route is generally shady. Pass The Wayside, the house with a history back to the Minute Men but famous now as the home of three literary families in the 19th century, including Louisa May Alcott, Nathaniel Hawthorne, and Margaret Sidney.

Continue past the Concord Museum to Monument Square, the heart of Concord. Concord is an amazingly tidy town, with immaculate houses and other buildings, many of which have historical significance.

If you want to see more revolutionary period historic sites, go north up Monument Street to North Bridge where it all started. Cross the bridge to see the famous Minute Man statue.

If you are ready for some food or a beverage, we can enthusiastically recommend the quaint 1716-vintage Colonial Inn at the west end of Monument Square. Food, drinks, and service are all excellent.

To get to the T commuter rail (a half-mile away), go south on Main Street. At the fork, take Sudbury Road to the left. It leads you to the station. Remember that commuter rail service can be quite infrequent so you should consult a timetable before leaving the Colonial Inn.

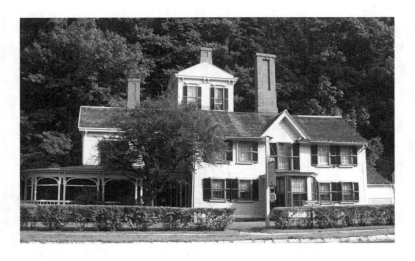

The Wayside—Home of Authors[2]

---

2   Photo courtesy National Parks Service.

Worcester: Elm Park

Distance	2.5+ miles
Comfort	Go a mile each way along the sidewalk of a relatively quiet, lightly trafficked street to get to and from the park. At the park, go around a comfortable half-mile paved loop trail as many times as you wish. Expect plenty of other people at the park, but not so many as to impede your use of the trail. Generally suitable for inline skating.
Attractions	Elm Park is very aesthetically attractive, including scenic lakes and bridges.
Convenience	Start and finish at City Hall in downtown Worcester. Elm Park is a mile from here via pleasant street sidewalks. The T commuter rail station is near City Hall.
Destination	Worcester Common in downtown Worcester, with nearby shops, restaurants, and pubs.

Worcester is the second-largest city in Massachusetts and the third-largest in New England. It is about 45 miles west of Boston and on a T commuter rail line, although you would probably not make the train trip from Boston just for an on-foot outing there.

Worcester is home to nine colleges and universities, and has various museums and cultural attractions. However, it has more the feel of a working class city than a college city. When out on foot, expect to see quite a lot of trash around and to encounter the occasional undesirable person. However, in most part, it is not threatening to the pedestrian, in daylight hours at least. There are quite a few hills so you have a good opportunity to keep fit if you exercise outdoors on foot. There are some marked trail systems and, according to the city's website, more planned.

We have checked out several on-foot ideas around Worcester and found two that meet our criteria, with qualifications.

The first goes from downtown to Elm Park, the park that is justifiably the city's pride and joy. This is a very pleasant on-foot route, and our only qualification is the shortness of the distance.

Start in Front Street at City Hall, across from the Worcester Common, at the city's heart. Go west to Main Street and find Elm Street, one

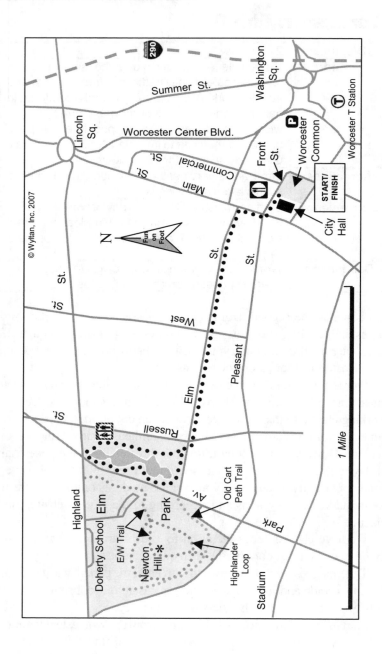

block to the north. Elm Street is a quiet, respectable, lightly trafficked street.

At the intersection with Russell Street you come to the eastern edge of Elm Park. The part of Elm Park on the east side of Park Avenue is one of the loveliest urban parks you will find anywhere. It has a beautiful lake system, complete with bridges, designed by no less than Frederick Law Olmsted. The bridges were reconstructed in 1985. The park is very popular with all types of residents, including runners, walkers, and families with children.

For your on-foot exercise, we suggest you simply do as many loops of the trail around the ponds as you wish (at roughly a half-mile per loop) and then return via Elm Street to downtown. (Add a mile each way between downtown and the park.)

VARIATION

The west part of Elm Park is entirely different in nature to the east part. Apart from the school and sporting fields on the northern edge, it comprises wilderness surrounding Newton Hill, with some marked hiking trails as shown on our map. So, if you feel like a little backwoods escape, then add an excursion over or around Newton Hill to your Elm Park outing. The reason we did not include this in our featured route is that we found this part of the park not very well maintained and surprisingly devoid of people on a weekend day, raising some comfort questions. You might be well advised to avoid Newton Hill if exercising without a companion.

If you want a food or beverage break after your exercise, there are many good choices in downtown Worcester. Our favorite is McFadden's Restaurant and Saloon at the intersection of Front Street and Commercial Street, near the Worcester Common.

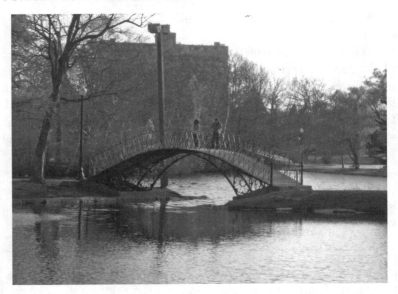

Olmsted's Influence is Unmistakable in Elm Park

Worcester: Green Hill Park

Distance	5.4 miles
Comfort	Roughly 3.6 miles along sidewalks of moderately busy streets getting to and from the park, with the remaining 1.8 miles on quiet but hilly paved trails inside the park. Expect plenty of other people around. Not very good for inline skating but it is possible.
Attractions	Green Hill Park is spacious and pleasant, with a good mix of community activity areas and wilderness. The route passes through the Massachusetts Vietnam Veterans' Memorial, which is extremely impressive and well worth visiting.
Convenience	Start and finish at City Hall in downtown Worcester. Green Hill Park is less than two miles from here via street sidewalks. The T commuter rail station is near City Hall.
Destination	Worcester Common in downtown Worcester, with nearby shops, restaurants, and pubs.

We introduced Worcester in the previous route. Our second Worcester route takes in the city's largest park, 480-acre Green Hill Park. This is an excellent place for on-foot exercise if you like some hilly terrain on good paved trails. Again, the route starts and finishes at City Hall and Worcester Common.

There are various ways to get to Green Hill Park from downtown. After exploring the options, we concluded that the best choice is to simply follow the most obvious main street sidewalks. (I discuss other options later.)

From City Hall, go up Main Street to the Lincoln Square traffic junction. Bear right onto Belmont Street. Use patience in getting through the various pedestrian crossings. Pass the beautiful Our Lady of Fatima Church and cross the Interstate. Follow the sidewalk of Belmont Street for about one mile. You come to Bell Pond on your right, at which point the route starts to become much more scenic. Continue to the Skyline Drive intersection and cross to the north side of Belmont Street.

Enter Green Hill Park and proceed up the hill. There are various foot trails through the park that you may wish to explore—check out

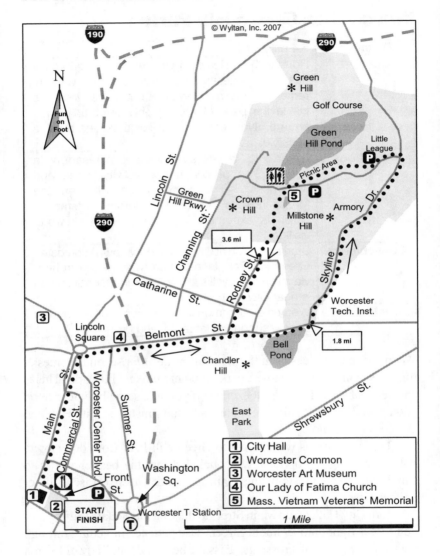

© Wyltan, Inc. 2007

the trail map sign at the entrance to the park. However, the simplest route is the paved path along Skyline Drive, a pleasant road with little traffic.

Go past the entrance to the Armory and up to where the main road does a sharp turn back to the left. Follow the road to the left past the little league field car park. You can optionally cut through that car park and follow a little footpath down towards Green Hill Pond. Continue to where the road comes close to the pond and passes the picnic area.

Here you come to the tastefully designed Massachusetts Vietnam Veterans' Memorial. This memorial, which occupies about four acres, is built around a small pond. It involves three main parts that are designated the Place of Flags, the Place of Words, and the Place of Names. The Place of Words, which is particularly moving, displays text from letters written home by some of the Soldiers, Sailors, Airmen and Marines who died in Vietnam. The Place of Names gives the names of all Massachusetts residents who died as a result of combat in Vietnam.

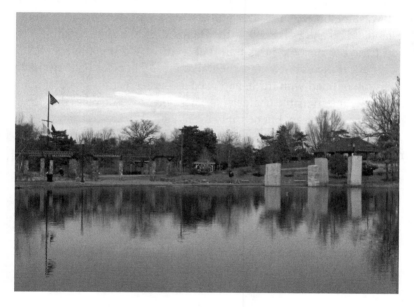

Massachusetts Vietnam Veterans' Memorial

While there are different ways out of the park from here, we suggest proceeding around the memorial and picking up the paved pedestrian and bike trail towards the south. This trail exits the park at the top end of Rodney Street, a quiet residential street. Rodney Street takes you to Belmont Street, which you can follow back to downtown, retracing your outbound route.

If you want a food or beverage break after your exercise, there are many good choices in downtown Worcester. Our favorite is McFadden's

Restaurant and Saloon at Front Street and Commercial Street near the Worcester Common.

* * * *

As I mentioned earlier, there are other ways to Green Hill Park, apart from simply following Belmont Street from Lincoln Square. Based on the website of the Regional Environmental Council of Central Massachusetts, the most interesting one appears to be a trail called "East Side Trail" from East Park (also known as Cristoforo Colombo Park). East Park is on Shrewsbury Street, a short walk from downtown via Washington Square. The trail passes through the reserve around Chandler Hill and Bell Pond, to the Belmont-Skyline intersection. Nola and I tried to negotiate this trail, but were very disappointed. While East Park is pleasant enough, the trail around Chandler Hill was badly overgrown, lined with trash, and used as the recreation space of some decidedly questionable characters. Therefore, I would class this "trail" as not just unpleasant but possibly even dangerous.

If you are going to take another route to Green Hill Park, I strongly recommend keeping to the streets.

Springfield: Forest Park

Distance	6.9 miles
Comfort	Roughly 3.6 miles along sidewalks of moderately busy streets getting to and from the park. The remaining 3.3 miles are on quiet trails inside the park, involving a mix of paved trails, earth trails, and park road sidewalks. Expect some other pedestrians around, including joggers. Not suitable for inline skating.
Attractions	Forest Park is a large, beautiful urban park, with a good mix of community activity areas and wilderness. There are attractive lakes, streams, and forest areas, with a well-maintained trail system.
Convenience	Start and finish at City Hall in downtown Springfield. Forest Park is less than two miles from here via street sidewalks.
Destination	Downtown Springfield, with plenty of shops, restaurants, pubs, and attractions that include the Basketball Hall of Fame, museums, and the Dr. Seuss National Memorial Sculpture Garden.

Springfield, 78 miles west of Boston, is the largest city in western Massachusetts. Springfield calls itself the "Crossroads of New England" but, since other places also claim that title, we cannot fully buy into it. However, Springfield certainly is at a major crossroads— the intersection of the Massachusetts Turnpike (Interstate 90) with the Connecticut River and Interstate 91.

More interestingly, Springfield has gained national prominence as the home of the NBA Basketball Hall of Fame. It is also recognized as the home of Theodore Seuss Geisel—Dr. Seuss.

Springfield is a pleasant city to visit. It has quite a few cultural attractions and a very helpful visitor information center. Also, the city obviously takes very seriously the need to provide and maintain on-foot trails. The only warning flag we have noticed is the very high violent crime statistic, of over 17 violent crimes per 1,000 residents (in 2005). While we have no particular cause for safety concerns in the part of the city covered in this route, you might want to keep that factor in mind whenever in Springfield.

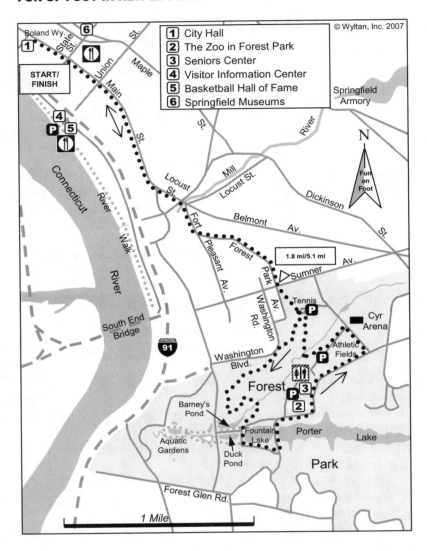

Forest Park, with 735 acres, is a very pleasant park. It is most famous for Bright Nights, a Christmas season tradition of decorating the trees with lights in the form of various characters, including those of Dr. Seuss. However, it is also an excellent place for every-day outdoor exercise.

Our route nominally starts at City Hall, in Main Street near Boland Way. Follow Main Street south, through a very ordinary part of the city, to the fork where Locust Street heads off to the left. Follow Locust Street across the river and then bear right into Fort Pleasant Avenue. From this point on, you are in a nice residential area with attractive homes. Go left into Forest Park Avenue and follow it to Sumner Avenue, at the top corner of Forest Park. Follow the foot trail entering the park from this street intersection.

There are several trails through Forest Park and we encourage you to explore, but detailed maps are hard to find. We found that even the map obtained from the park's vehicle entrance booth (a block east of where we entered on foot) is not enormously helpful. For our featured route, we therefore decided to stick to trails that are easy to navigate and generally amenable to running more so than just hiking.

On entering the park at the Forest Park-Sumner intersection, there is a wide, unpaved, well-used trail from the corner going straight in at an angle to a parking lot at the end of a dead-end road (there are tennis courts on the left). At the far right corner of the asphalt area, there is a paved non-vehicle trail heading off to the right and, after a short distance, a well-used earth trail taking off perpendicularly from it to the left. We suggest taking the paved trail initially. (Later we return via that earth trail.)

The paved trail takes you to the edge of Washington Road where it turns into Washington Boulevard. Keep inside the park, bearing left onto the major unpaved trail. Follow the main trail (there are some smaller side-trails). Continue to where you notice a road down the ridge to the right and a lake straight ahead. Take the main trail to the left that brings you around to a little bridge over the stream, Meadow Brook. Then bear right to the road and the more populated area where Barney's Pond, Duck Pond, and Fountain Lake all meet.

Cross the paved causeway between Duck Pond and Fountain Lake, and continue following the paved road around to the left. You come to a T-intersection. Go left back past the lakes and up to the more heavily used road.

VARIATION

There are foot trails around Porter Lake, but they are steep, narrow, uncared-for, and generally for the more adventurous hiker.

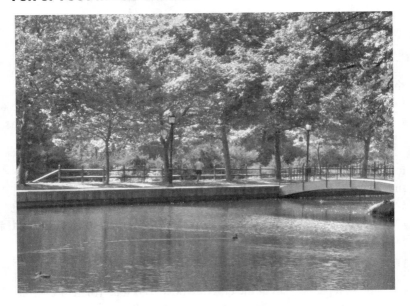

The Forest Park Lakes

Bear right, with the zoo on your left. Follow the paved sidewalk around to the zoo entrance and the Senior Center. There are restrooms at the Senior Center. Follow the paved footpath along the road and around the sporting fields. You come to the main ball field grandstand. Go left around that, following the road.

A paved pedestrian trail takes off to the right. Follow it down to its end. Cross the stream and follow the main trail (now an earth trail) up. It takes you through forest back to the paved trail near the dead-end road at the tennis courts, where we were earlier.

To return downtown, retrace your steps to Main Street and continue to City Hall. Another good destination is the Basketball Hall of Fame. To go there, follow Union Street to the left off Main Street, and proceed under the Interstate to the Hall of Fame. If you are ready for a food and beverage break, there is an excellent establishment, Max's Tavern, adjacent to the Hall of Fame.

If you want to see other Springfield sights, such as the museums or the Dr. Seuss National Memorial Sculpture Garden (adjacent to the museums), drop into the helpful Visitor Center, one short block northwest of the Hall of Fame, for more information.

* * * *

Another interesting on-foot exercise option in Springfield is the River Walk along the Connecticut River, reachable via the bridge over the tracks near the Visitor Center and the Hall of Fame. This project, unfortunately, is still incomplete. We would love to have found a way to Forest Park via this trail but, regrettably, that is just not possible today.

Other Routes

Amherst is a lovely college town in western Massachusetts, north of Springfield. It has some good on-foot exercise routes. The **Norwottuck Rail Trail** is a particularly pleasant trail, linking Amherst with **Northampton**. There is a connector trail to it from the University of Massachusetts Amherst campus. This trail is very popular with both joggers and cyclists. However, it does not easily build a circular loop. You have to go out-and-back to whatever point you choose on the former rail line.[3]

Amherst also has a series of on-foot trails called **Literary Trails**, dedicated to the various famous writers who have lived in the town. It is possible to build some loops using those literary trails in combination with the Norwottuck Rail Trail and we tried that but failed to find really good routes. The trails were, all too often, narrow, steep, and overgrown. You would need to be a sturdy backwoods hiker to appreciate them. On one trail we tried, we almost stepped on two snakes along the way—that in itself caused Nola to veto any thought of featuring such trails in this book.

The **Bay Circuit Trail** is an ambitious off-road trail project intended to link 50 cities and towns in a 200-mile ring around Boston. It will start at Newburyport on the North Shore and end at Duxbury on the South Shore. It is early days for this project but watch for the opportunity to build some good Fun-on-Foot routes in the future based on the Bay Circuit Trail.

Another ambitious trail project is the **Blackstone River Bikeway**, extending from **Worcester** in the north to Providence, Rhode Island, in the south. The Massachusetts section, 28 miles in length, is being progressively constructed. It will link several historic mill villages along the Blackstone River. Near the Worcester end, this trail will also have an access path to the **Broad Meadow Brook Wildlife Sanctuary**, which has its own trail system. This might lead to an interesting Fun-on-Foot route out from Worcester in the future.[4]

The **Connecticut River Walk and Bikeway** is an interesting project linking the centers of **Holyoke**, **Chicopee**, **West Springfield**, **Springfield**, and **Agawam** via trails along the Connecticut River. Parts are complete but major pieces are yet to be filled in.

3   See: http://www.mass.gov/dcr/parks/central/nwrt.htm
4   See: http://www.blackstoneriverbikeway.com

Newburyport is a picturesque little coastal city at the mouth of the Merrimack River at the top end of the Massachusetts North Shore. It is reachable from Boston by Commuter Rail. Unfortunately there are no trails of note around the center. There is an excellent set of on-foot trails about three miles west of Newburyport in **Maudslay State Park**.[5] Nola and I tried hard to find a way to sensibly link this park and the city center into an attractive on-foot route but failed in that. Also, about four miles east of Newburyport is the beach area of **Plum Island** where you can run on the beach.[6] Again, we failed to find a nice on-foot link between there and the city center. If you are around Newburyport and want some on-foot exercise, the best option is to drive to Maudslay State Park or to Plum Island, park your vehicle, and do a nice on-foot loop there.

The city of **Northampton**, home to Smith College, has a 1.75-mile paved rail trail to Look Memorial Park, a local park with facilities for all ages. It is less than a mile to the start of the trail from downtown, via Route 9 and State Street.

Plymouth is an interesting place, of great historic significance, and on a Commuter Rail line. Do not fail to come here to see the Plymouth Rock and the Pilgrim Hall Museum. Unfortunately, there is not much in the way of on-foot routes around Plymouth. The best trails around here are in the **Myles Standish State Forest**, several miles southwest.[7] That is a fine place to drive to and hike or run, but is not convenient to any city or town.

We described an excellent trail in **Rockport** but there are other on-foot opportunities near here as well. In particular, less than three miles north of town is **Halibut Point Reservation and State Park**, one of the most scenic locations on the ocean shore. Unfortunately there is no convenient way to get there other than driving, so we shall leave that exercise to you.[8]

* * * *

---

5   See: http://www.mass.gov/dcr/parks/northeast/maud.htm
6   Beaches here are often closed from spring into July to protect the piping plover nesting areas. Also, access to the area is restricted during the annual deer hunt.
7   See: http://www.mass.gov/dcr/parks/southeast/mssf.htm
8   See: http://www.mass.gov/dcr/parks/northeast/halb.htm

Massachusetts has an unlimited number of pleasant places to get out on-foot. I believe we have covered some of the best ones—at least those close to the more highly populated areas. We shall leave the more remote regions of the state to you to develop your own Fun-on-Foot ideas.

Let us now move on to the other New England States, progressing from the more populous to the less populous states...

Constitution State: Connecticut

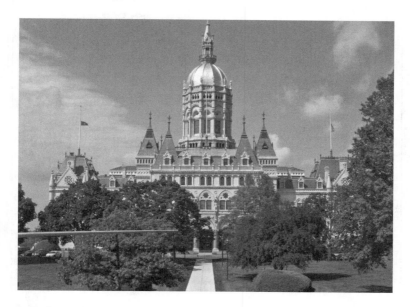

Connecticut, the fifth state to join the union and the third smallest state, always feels a little different to the other New England states. On one hand, it shares the qualities of those states, such as plenty of forested backwoods terrain and many miles of scenic coastline. Also, like the other states, it has all sorts of special little places to hide away or to share the company of others in select, beautiful, localities.

On the other hand, Connecticut sometimes seems to be more an extension nursery of that dark center of the south, New York City. Some out-of-Connecticut New Englanders think of Connecticut as a massive

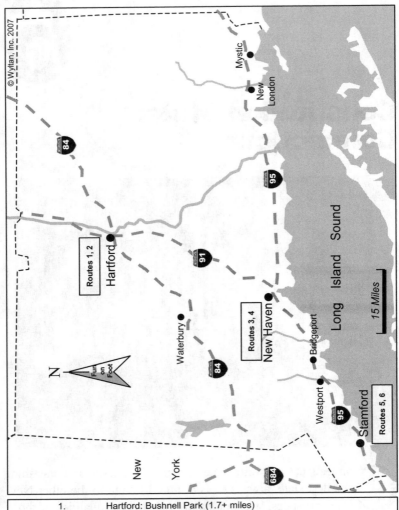

1.	Hartford: Bushnell Park (1.7+ miles)
2.	Hartford: Connecticut River Loop (3.7 miles)
3.	New Haven: Downtown and Campus Loop (2.9 miles)
4.	New Haven: East Rock Park (3.3 miles)
5.	Stamford: Downtown and Scalzi Park (3.3+ miles)
6.	Stamford: Cove Island and Cummings Parks (6.3 miles)

Connecticut Featured Routes

highway system that connects the heart of New England to the dark center and beyond.

When applying our Fun on Foot model to Connecticut, we took the usual approach of focusing on the major population centers and places that attract many visitors. Connecticut has several sizable urban centers, and our research produced mixed results. Most of the state's larger centers have a highly industrial background that tends to lower their appeal. In some cases, we found little in the way of outdoor exercise routes worthy of mentioning in this book. In other places, we were pleasantly surprised by the extent to which communities are driving forward programs to improve their downtown centers and make on-foot exercise accessible to and friendly for everyone.

We ended up focusing on three urban centers: the state capital, Hartford; the home of Yale, New Haven; and the big city of the southwest, Stamford. We feature six routes in these cities, and discuss other places at the end.

Hartford: Bushnell Park

Distance	1.7+ miles
Comfort	This route is along street sidewalks and paths around and through a popular urban park. Expect plenty of other people around, including joggers. Parts of the route can be crowded on a busy summer weekend or holiday. Not suitable for inline skating.
Attractions	A beautiful park containing an outstanding collection of tree varieties, the majestic Connecticut State House, and the Gothic-architecture Soldiers and Sailors Memorial Arch.
Convenience	Start and end at the Civic Center, close to major downtown hotels and restaurants. This location is easily reached by free shuttle from the Connecticut Convention Center and other parts of downtown.
Destination	Downtown Hartford, with shops, restaurants, and pubs.

Hartford has an impressive history. Its background includes being the state capital of the fifth state, the insurance capital of the nation, and the home of Mark Twain while he wrote his most famous works. Despite those credentials, downtown Hartford has for many years been considered a place to prudently avoid. It certainly does not have a reputation that engenders enthusiasm for exercising outdoors.

I am happy to report, however, that that situation is rapidly changing. Hartford has taken tremendous steps to restore its downtown core to a state attractive to visitors. There are new hotels, shops, restaurants, and bars. The streets are clean, and there is a free shuttle bus around downtown. There is a Welcome Center for visitors.

Admittedly, there is some way to go: The shuttle does not run on Sundays and the Welcome Center is closed on weekends. However, I am sure that the powers-that-be will soon work out how dumb those policies are, and what it really takes to make visitors feel comfortable.

Most importantly, the city is reaching the point where exercising outdoors is a pleasant and comfortable activity. Hartford has hosted a marathon for several years, but now running, jogging, and walking are starting to become part of the every-day community agenda.

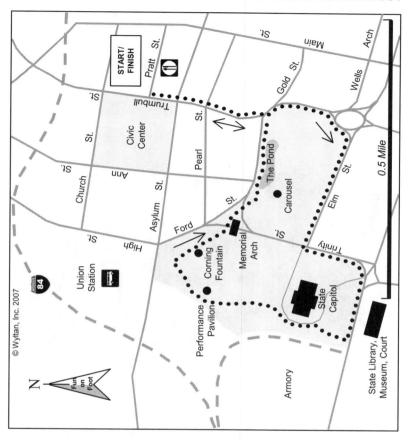

We found two nice routes to recommend. This first route is a simple one, and shorter than we like. However, it covers what is unquestionably the most popular jogging place in the city, and is a great first on-foot outing for anyone visiting Hartford.

When it comes to parks, Bushnell Park is Hartford's pride and joy. It was designed in 1861 by Jacob Weidenmann, under contract to the city and on the recommendation of Frederick Law Olmsted, a Hartford native.

Our route nominally starts and finishes by the Civic Center, in Trumbull Street, which is arguably the heart of downtown. Go south down Trumbull Street and cross the street at the end to enter the eastern end of Bushnell Park. Proceed around the perimeter of the park clockwise. On reaching Trinity Street, cross the street and go left around the perimeter of the west part of the park. Work your way around the 1876-vintage State Capitol, keeping close to its western side. Continue into the green and spacious park proper.

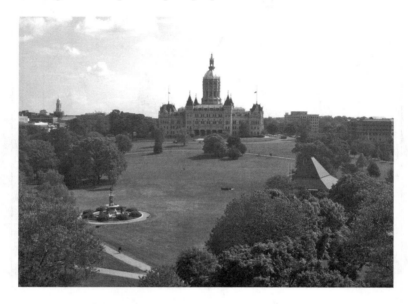

Bushnell Park West—Corning Fountain and State Capitol

Go past the Performance Pavilion, and follow the trail around to the marble and stone Corning Fountain, erected by John Corning of Corning Glass Works in 1899. Continue on to the Soldiers and Sailors Memorial Arch, dedicated in 1886 to honor the 4,000 Hartford citizens who served in the Civil War, and the 400 who died for the Union.

Cross the street and proceed along the edge of The Pond. Divert to see the 1914-vintage carousel if that interests you. Continue to Trumbull Street, where you first entered the park, and then return to the Civic Center. If you want some more distance, do a few loops around the east side of the park (about three-quarters of a mile loop) first.

If you want a food and beverage break, there are several good places in and near Pratt Street, where our route nominally terminates. We particularly enjoyed Vaughan's Public House, a quaint Irish pub with an enticing black and gold facade in Pratt Street, and the City Steam Brewery in Main Street near Pratt.

Hartford: Connecticut River Loop

Distance	3.7 miles
Comfort	Roughly one mile is along street sidewalks getting to and from the river and the remainder is on shared pedestrian/bicycle trails. These trails are mostly, but not completely, paved. Expect ample other people around, including other on-foot exercisers. OK for inline skating in parts but not overall.
Attractions	A trail through an attractive river setting, with some excellent views of the downtown skyline. An escape from the hustle and bustle of the city.
Convenience	Start and end at the Civic Center, close to major downtown hotels and restaurants. This location is easily reached by free shuttle from the Connecticut Convention Center and other parts of downtown.
Destination	Downtown Hartford, with shops, restaurants, and pubs.

The river is one area that Hartford has taken major steps to clean up and turn into an attractive place for recreation and on-foot exercise. Unfortunately, the year that we explored the riverbanks, there had been substantial flooding in the spring and the area had not fully recovered by the middle of summer. I guess that is a risk that will always be present.

Nevertheless, we found one very enjoyable loop route—a river loop between the Founders Bridge and the Charter Oak Bridge. We also looked into possible routes upstream from the Founders Bridge and we discuss that later. One thing that delighted us about the route described below is that, despite the less-than-ideal conditions, we met many nice, friendly, welcoming locals along the way, taking part in activities ranging from jogging, to fishing, to family picnicking. That raised our confidence in this route enormously.

As with our previous route, we nominally start and finish by the Civic Center, in Trumbull Street, near the best pubs and restaurants. Go south down Trumbull Street and turn left into Asylum Street. Continue straight towards the river where you run into the pedestrian plaza over Interstate 91 called Riverfront Plaza.

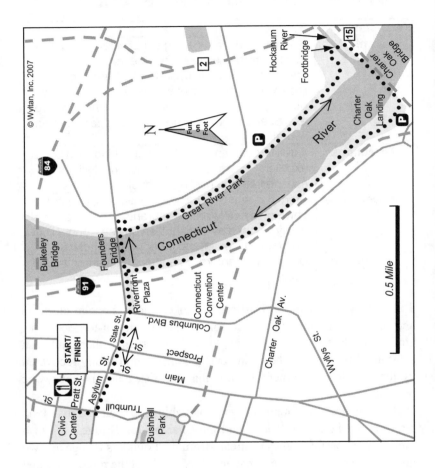

Go through Riverfront Plaza and cross Founders Bridge over the river, via a very wide pedestrian sidewalk. Adjacent traffic is typically light. On the other side, go down the disabled ramp and then the steps down to the riverbank. Take the trail to the left, downstream. Enter Great River Park. There is a very pleasant, well-maintained, paved trail here. Continue southward until you are forced to go a short distance away from the river to cross the tributary Hockanum River via a foot-bridge.

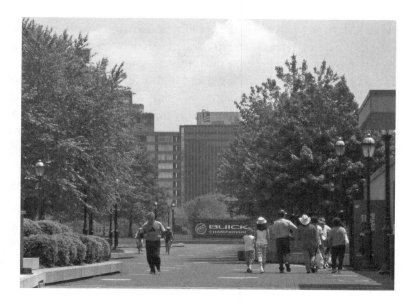

Riverfront Plaza

Mount the steps up to the sidewalk of the Charter Oak Bridge and cross that bridge. The views from here are excellent. On the other side, go down the steps and enter the park called Charter Oak Landing. This is a nice, relaxed park with playgrounds and picnic spots, popular with local families on weekends.

Go to the north end of Charter Oak Landing and find the trail up the river towards downtown Hartford. The trails are rougher here than on the other side of the river, but there are active plans to improve them. You come to the outlet of a now-hidden river called Park River. Work your way around this and continue on the trail until you are back to urban civilization at Riverfront Plaza.

Retrace you original route to the Pratt Street area and enjoy a snack or beverage at one of those great restaurant/pubs.

* * * *

I said earlier we looked at the river trail upstream of the Founders Bridge. Frankly, we were a little disappointed. There is a nice park, called Riverside Park, which can be reached by following a trail upstream a half-mile and beyond from Riverfront Plaza on the city side of the river. However, the on-foot access from that park back to the city side of Interstate 91 frustrated us enormously. There is a pedestrian overpass bridge over the Interstate, connecting with the end of Pequot Street. Significantly, the end of that bridge is quite close to the Connecticut Expo Center (not to be confused with the Connecticut Convention Center), making it potentially important for visitors staying near there. Unfortunately, the run-down nature of the area around that bridge, and the questionable people frequenting that area, caused us to write it off our recommendations. Hopefully the Hartford powers-that-be will fix that problem soon, giving us another valuable Fun-on-Foot route.

New Haven: Downtown and Campus Loop

Distance	2.9 miles
Comfort	This route is entirely along street sidewalks in and near the Yale campus. Expect plenty of other people around, and there is a risk of crowding in some spots. Not suitable for inline skating.
Attractions	The outstanding architecture of the Yale buildings. This route gives you a tour of Yale in combination with an on-foot exercise outing. New Haven has a very impressive city center.
Convenience	Start and end at the intersection of College and Chapel Streets, at the New Haven Green. This is the heart of the city and is close to hotels and restaurants, and attractions such as the Yale University Art Gallery.
Destination	Downtown New Haven, close to museums and Yale sights and destinations. Restaurants and pubs are close by, mostly around Chapel Street.

New Haven, known as Elm City, is the second-largest city in Connecticut (Bridgeport is the largest). The city's main claim to fame today is the home of ivy-league Yale University. New Haven has a long and austere history, stretching back to its founding in 1638. Among other things, it claims to be the birthplace of American football and the Frisbee, and the location of the first telephone exchange and telephone directory.

New Haven's city center is a very impressive place, thanks to the amazing collection of architectural masterpieces provided by Yale. Being very compact, it is also a very pleasant place to tour on foot.

Some of New Haven's suburban areas are a lot less prosperous than the city core, so you might want to bear that in mind when wandering around the wider city.

We feature two New Haven routes. The first is a simple loop that takes in some of the high points of the Yale campus scene. If you are a visitor to the city or a returning alumnus, it is a perfect introduction to today's New Haven. The second route is more demanding athletically, and can be combined with the first if you wish.

This route starts and finishes at the intersection of Chapel Street and College Street. Not only is this at the New Haven Green, the historical city center, but it also happens to be very close to the city's best restaurants and pubs, should you feel like a food or beverage break afterwards.

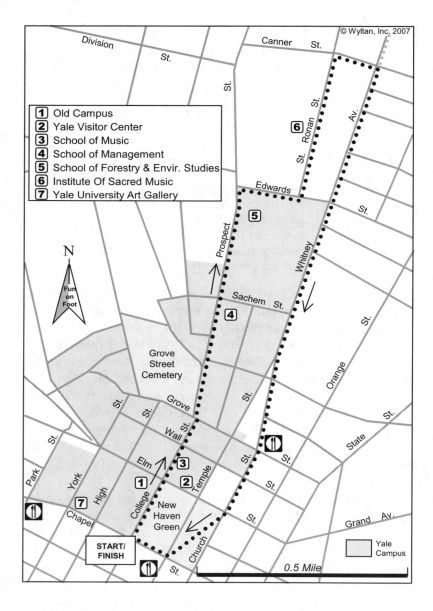

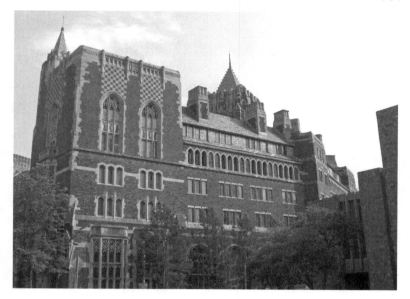

Yale's Imposing Architecture

Head north up College Street, past the old campus area. Cross Elm Street—to your right in Elm Street is the Yale visitor center, where you can pick up a campus map. Pass the School of Music on your right. At Grove Street, College Street ends—continue straight ahead into Prospect Street. Pass the Grove Street Cemetery on your left. Admire the Yale architecture here and elsewhere along this route.

Continue up Prospect Street past the School of Management and the School of Forestry and Environmental Studies. Turn right into Edwards Street. This is the highest point, elevation-wise, of this route. Turn left into St. Ronan Street. You pass some very classy Yale residences and the Institute of Sacred Music on this stretch. Turn right on Canner Street and go on to Whitney Avenue.

VARIATION

At this point you can tack on our other New Haven route, going out of the urban center and into the more strenuous terrain of East Rock Park. See details in the next route description.

Turn right heading south on Whitney Avenue. Continue to where the road forks, with the Yale campus on your right. Take the left fork and continue to Grove Street. On the left you pass Anna Liffey's Irish Pub, one of our recommended food/beverage stops.

Whitney Avenue now runs into Church Street. Continue down to Elm Street and the northeast corner of New Haven Green. Go diagonally through the Lower Green (the eastern section) to the Chapel and Temple intersection. The route ends a block west at Chapel and College.

If you have the time, take a stroll through the Upper Green (the western section) and admire its three 19th-century churches. The Yale University Art Gallery, with a collection of over 100,000 pieces of art from ancient Egypt through to the present day, is also nearby, in Chapel Street at York Street.

If you need a food or beverage stop, there are many restaurants around this part of Chapel Street, in particular several Asian choices. We fell back to our usual preference—the Irish Pub. Our favorite is The Playwright, a short walk down Temple Street from Chapel Street. It is a very impressive Irish pub. Its interior, imported from Ireland, is taken from an old church. We can also recommend O'Sullivans on Chapel Street near Park Street and Anna Liffey's at 17 Whitney Avenue.

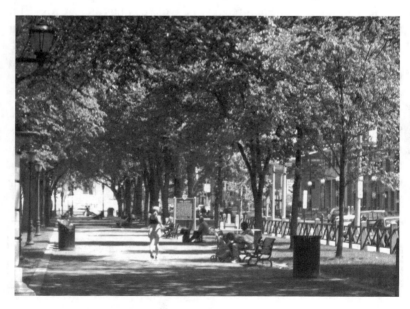

New Haven Green

New Haven: East Rock Park

Distance	3.3 miles
Comfort	1.8 miles of this route are along unpaved pedestrian trails, with the remaining 1.5 miles along good street sidewalks. There are a couple of steeper and rougher parts, but most of the route is runnable. Expect plenty of other people around, but no crowds. Not suitable for inline skating.
Attractions	Excellent views of the whole New Haven area from the top of East Rock. An enjoyable escape from the urban world into the world of nature. Cross a covered bridge and, if interested, visit the Eli Whitney Museum.
Convenience	Start and end at the intersection of Whitney Avenue and Canner Street, about 1.5 miles from central New Haven by foot (as per our previous route). Alternatively, you can drive and park near here.
Destination	Plan on tacking on the return 1.5 miles to down-town New Haven, close to museums, the Yale campus, restaurants, and pubs.

Our second New Haven route is very different to the first, in that it is more a mountain-hiking trek than a city street walk or jog. While it has a couple of steeper and rougher spots, it is not very difficult though, and the athletic person could run almost all of it. Even Nola and I hiked it easily in just over an hour. It is well worth it for the outstanding views.

We nominally start and finish at the intersection of Whitney Avenue and Canner Street, at the extreme point of our first route. Our idea is that you link up these two routes to give you an excellent 6.2-mile outing. You have lots of flexibility though, and can drive and park near the start point if you wish.

Go one block north up Whitney Avenue to Cold Spring Street. Turn right and go two blocks to College Woods Park. This is a popular park for family picnics and recreation. There is a ranger station there but do not rely on it being open.

Go through the park to Orange Street on its eastern side. Follow Orange Street across the bridge over the Mill River. Bear right and

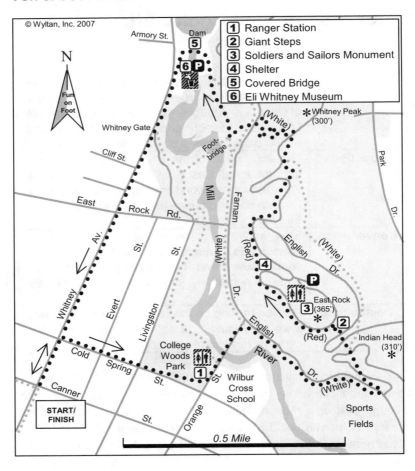

© Wyltan, Inc. 2007

N

Fun on Foot

1	Ranger Station
2	Giant Steps
3	Soldiers and Sailors Monument
4	Shelter
5	Covered Bridge
6	Eli Whitney Museum

Armory St.

Dam **5**

6 P

Whitney Peak (300')

(White)

Whitney Gate

Cliff St.

Foot-bridge

Mill

Farnam

East Rock Rd.

Av.

St.

St.

(White)

(Red)

English Dr.

(White)

4

Whitney

Evert

Livingston

P

East Rock (365')

3 ✻

2

Park Dr.

Cold

Spring St.

College Woods Park

1

Wilbur Cross School

(Red)

English River

Dr.

Indian Head (310') ✻

Canner

START/ FINISH

St.

Orange St.

Sports Fields

(White)

0.5 Mile

pick up the foot trail tracking the road. Note the white rectangular trail markers on this trail. This park has a system of colored trail blazes, and we use both white-blazed and red-blazed trails in this route.

When you come to the ball fields, find the path heading across the road and continuing uphill on the other side. It continues to have the white markers.

You reach a trail junction where a side trail takes off to the left up steps. This trail has red triangular markers. Follow this red trail up the steps. If you chose to keep to the main (white-blazed) trail you would still link up with us later but would miss out on the best scenic views.

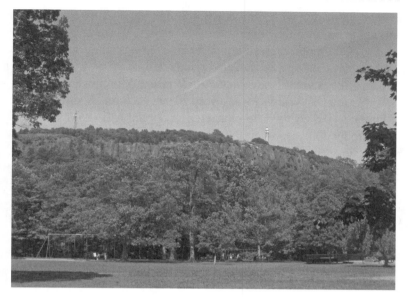

East Rock Towering Above College Woods Park

The steps, known as the Giant Steps, are many and steep. This is a somewhat strenuous climb, but we encountered some people running up. The payout for this exercise comes at the top of the steps, where you emerge at the top of a steep ridge with an outstanding view of New Haven city and beyond.

This is the top of East Rock. There is an excellent view as far as Long Island Sound and beyond to Long Island on a clear day. It is a popular place, so expect plenty of people around, especially on a summer weekend. (Most of them drove up, missing out on the exercise benefits you are gaining.) We even encountered an ice cream vendor up there, and could not resist his wares.

Admire the 112-foot-high Soldiers and Sailors Monument. Erected in 1887, this monument honors New Haven residents who gave their lives in the Revolutionary War, the War of 1812, the Mexican War, and the Civil War.

From the East Rock summit, find the continuing red-marked trail following the ridge northward. The trail is a bit rough in parts, but if necessary you can switch to the nearby road to bypass difficult parts. Eventually the red trail re-connects with the white trail. Keep bearing left and follow the white trail down from the ridge. In due course you will come close to the bank of the Mill River. There is a footbridge nearby, but a more interesting option is to go upstream on the trail a short distance and find the covered bridge.

Cross the covered bridge to the Eli Whitney Museum and Whitney Water Center. Eli Whitney was a very talented person. A Yale graduate in the late 18th century, he pioneered important aspects of industrial mass production. He is attributed with inventing the cotton gin, and built a gun-manufacturing factory here in New Haven. That factory is now the Eli Whitney museum.

Follow Whitney Avenue south, past the Whitney Gate of East Rock Park. This is quite a popular area for local joggers. Continue south to Canner Street where our route started. If tacking this route onto our first New Haven route, continue back to downtown, and enjoy a good pub, restaurant, museum, or other destination there.

Stamford: Downtown and Scalzi Park

Distance	3.3+ miles
Comfort	Most of this route is along good street sidewalks, with some stretches along paved paths in city parks. To extend the distance beyond 3.3 miles, you can add loops of the pleasant paved track in Scalzi Park. Expect plenty of other people around, but crowds are unlikely. Not suitable for inline skating.
Attractions	See much of the city core. Scalzi Park is very pleasant and has the most popular jogging track in Stamford.
Convenience	Start and end at the intersection of Atlantic Street and Main Street at the center of the city, close to downtown hotels and the Amtrak station.
Destination	Downtown Stamford, with its many shops, restaurants, and pubs.

The fact that you see more Yankees caps than Red Sox caps in Stamford suggests that this city is more a nursery suburb for New York than it is a part of the New England core. However, in recent years, Stamford has grown into much more than an extension of the New York tentacles—it is now a major business center in its own right. Along with this growth have come several quality hotels, restaurants, entertainment venues, and a major increase in its visitor appeal overall.

Concerns that once existed over crime here have seriously diminished. The FBI figures show a very modest crime rate of less than three violent crimes per 1,000 inhabitants (in 2005). The city's website proudly boasts of double-digit decreases in the crime rate each year of the current Mayor's term. I think I can believe this, and so salute the Mayor. Stamford is now a really lovely city to visit.

For visitors staying in downtown Stamford, we have laid out a simple 3.3-mile route that might prove valuable for a morning jog before breakfast. It also serves to get you to Scalzi Park, which is the center of the city's on-foot athletic activities.

We nominally start and end at the city's heart, Old Town Hall near Veterans Park, where Main Street meets Atlantic Street. This is handy to all downtown hotels. Follow Main Street westward to the river and cross over the disused road bridge. Turn right following the riverbank

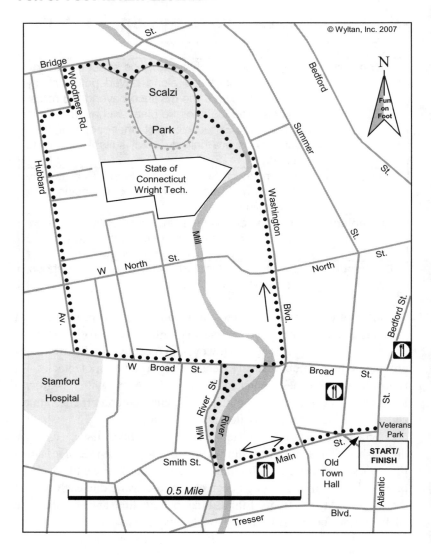

© Wyltan, Inc. 2007

into the very pleasant park here. Take the paved trail up to Broad Street. Cross the river and Broad Street here, and then continue northward on the wide pedestrian sidewalk of Washington Boulevard. You come to the south end of Scalzi Park. Cross the footbridge into the park proper. Go around the park loop either direction. Exit at the northwest corner of the park onto the edge of Bridge Street.

VARIATION
Add in as many loops as you want of the popular, roughly half-mile circuit in Scalzi Park.

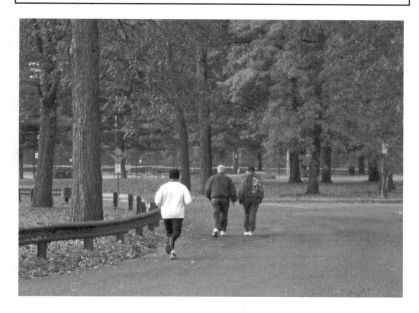

The Popular Loop in Pretty Scalzi Park

From Bridge Street take the first left into Woodmere Road. This is a very pleasant little tree-lined street with beautiful houses and a sidewalk (not all streets around here have that luxury, but we try to stick to those that do). Woodmere leads you to Hubbard Avenue, where you head to the left. Hubbard is another very impressive residential street, with houses having a variety of classy architectures. Go down Hubbard to W Broad Street, by the Stamford Hospital, where you turn left. We do not recommend heading west from here since the quality of the neighborhoods declines substantially.

Follow W Broad Street back to Mill River Street and the park you passed through earlier. Turn right onto the park trail back to the Main Street bridge. Cross that bridge, and follow Main Street back to the center of downtown.

If you are interested in a food or drink destination, there are many great choices in Stamford, a short walk from our route's endpoint. They are mainly clustered in three areas:

1. Around the west part of Main Street (which we traversed in this route);

2. Up Summer Street between Main Street and Broad Street and further north from there; and

3. In Bedford Street one block east of Summer Street and north of Broad Street.

We have checked out several places, especially the Irish pubs. Our favorite Irish pubs were Tiernan's in Main Street, and Tigin and the Temple Bar, both in Bedford Street.

Stamford: Cove Island and Cummings Parks

Distance	6.3 miles
Comfort	4.5 miles of this route are along street sidewalks, with the remaining 1.8 miles on well-maintained paths in the parks. Expect plenty of other people around. Not suitable for inline skating, but there is an excellent one-mile loop trail designed for bikes and inline skaters in Cove Island Park.
Attractions	Two very pleasant seaside parks with scenic ocean views, beaches, and good jogging trails.
Convenience	Start and end at the intersection of Atlantic Street and Main Street at the center of the city, close to downtown hotels and the Amtrak station.
Destination	Downtown Stamford, with its many shops, restaurants, and pubs.

Stamford has one place that stands out as an extremely enjoyable place for on-foot exercise—Cove Island Park. This is a well cared-for park with excellent facilities, trails, a beach, and scenic views of both Long Island Sound and a major estuary known as Holly Pond. It is very popular with all Stamford residents interested in outdoor exercise or just some fresh air. While most locals would drive here, it is just over two miles on-foot from the city center through respectable (albeit not beautiful) neighborhoods. Furthermore, with a minor diversion, the route from downtown to Cove Island can also take in Cummings Park, Stamford's other major seaside park. Therefore, we decided to construct a route from downtown that visits both parks.

Start from Veterans Park and find your way through the shopping mall to its eastern exit—this is maybe the most challenging part of the route, especially if you are a shopaholic.

Find Main Street at its intersection with Greyrock Place. Follow Main Street eastward. Cross Tresser Boulevard at the traffic light and enter Elm Street, keeping to its right side and heading toward the Interstate-95 underpass. Go under the Interstate and the rail tracks and follow Elm Street to its intersection with Cove Road and Shippan Avenue. This part of the route is not all beautiful but has some attractive

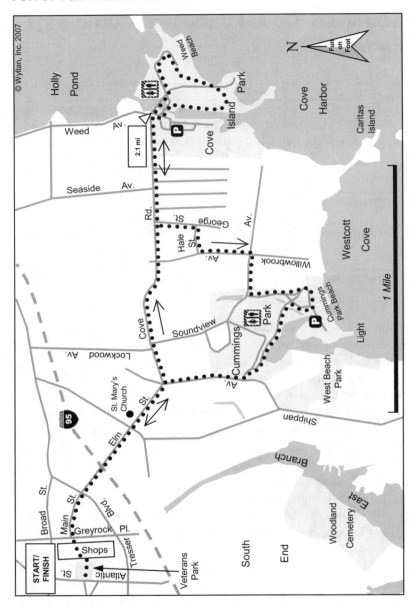

parts, such as the majestic Saint Mary's Catholic Church. In our experience, there were plenty of other people around and no warning signs of major safety concerns.

Bear left following Cove Road 1.2 miles to the parking lot of Cove Island Park. Cross the footbridge and you are in one of Connecticut's loveliest urban recreational areas. There are various trails here, including unpaved trails for on-footers and a paved one-mile circuit intended for bikes and inline skating. Admire the beach and, if you are here in summer, take a beach break. In our mileage, we assumed doing 1.1 miles here, but running multiple loops is a quite common practice and I would encourage that.

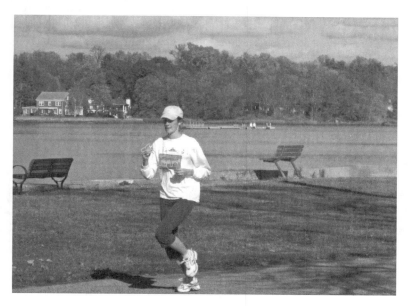

Jogging in Cove Island Park

Leave the park the same way you entered. Unfortunately there is no way out along the shore to the south, since that part is private land. That area includes the access road to Caritas Island, recognized as one of the most exclusive private islands in the world.

Go back along Cove Road to George Street on the left. Turn left into George Street, right into Hale Street, and then left into Willowbrook Avenue. These are all nice, quiet residential streets.

Turn right into Soundview Avenue and follow it into Cummings Park. This is a large 79-acre park, with many sporting facilities, a beach at its southern edge, and a lot of open green space. Entering the park via Soundview Avenue gives you several choices as to which route to follow through the park. For the shortest route, leave the road and cross the fields going straight ahead, picking up paved trails and sidewalks as you find them. Keep going generally westward and find the exit road from the park onto Shippan Avenue. There are many other options, however, including passing by the beach to the south. We shall leave this decision to you. For mileage purposes, we assume you travel 0.7 mile in Cummings Park.

Exit Cummings Park onto Shippan Avenue, and head to the right to the Elm Street intersection. Follow Elm Street back to downtown, retracing the start of the route. Food and beverage destinations downtown are discussed in our previous route description.

Other Routes

If I am accused of not covering enough routes in Connecticut, based on its population, I must plead guilty. Connecticut is the second-largest New England state population-wise, with roughly half the population of Massachusetts. However, our route selection process focuses on the main population areas and, in the case of Connecticut, we were a little disappointed with the suitability of its larger cities for on-foot exercise. Following are some suggestions for on-foot routes not covered above.

Bridgeport is Connecticut's largest city. However, it is very much an industrial city and is not a significant travel destination. It has relatively few hotels, few downtown attractions, and many questionable areas for pedestrians. It does, however, have one beautiful asset for pedestrians— **Seaside Park**. This park, which stretches two miles along the shore, offers sporting fields, beaches, and scenic views of Long Island Sound. It is quite popular with locals, but they warn you to stay away near dark. Seaside Park is adjacent to the University of Bridgeport campus, so it is a tremendous resource for students there. The biggest problem from the Fun-on-Foot perspective is that all routes from the city center to Seaside Park pass through less-than-pleasant and somewhat questionable areas. Therefore, we did not feature this route, although you might like to drive to the park for a run on a nice summer day.

Another nice area for on-foot exercise in Bridgeport is **Beardsley Park**, up the Pequondock River about three miles from downtown.[1] This park is also home to Connecticut's premier zoo, Beardsley Zoo. You can run a pleasant two-mile loop within this park. Unfortunately, it is not conveniently reachable on-foot from downtown. Another area I have heard recommended is the **Black Rock** area, west of the city center.

In our second **Hartford** route description, I mentioned the trail north from Riverfront Plaza to **Riverfront Park**. While this did not make our quality cut for this book, please explore and enjoy it. Further out of Hartford, about six miles to the west, there is an extensive trail system at **West Hartford Reservoir**. You can access this area from Farmington Avenue (Route 4). There is a paved three-mile walking loop, closed to traffic, plus some light hiking trails that are suitable for running.

---

1   See: www.beardsleyzoo.org

The pleasant town of **Greenwich**, west of Stamford, has a 60-acre park, **Bruce Park**, easily accessible on foot from the center of town. Among other recreational activities, there are some short jogging and walking trails in this park.[2]

Both **Monroe** and **Trumbull** have sections of trail complete along the **Housatonic Railbed**, and plans are in place to link these and eventually fill out an 18.5-mile trail along this rail-bed from the downtown Bridgeport transportation center through Trumbull and Monroe to the edge of **Newtown**.[3]

Mystic is a lovely area which many people visit for its tourist attractions, notably the historic Mystic Seaport. There are plenty of opportunities for on-foot exercise along the streets here, but no trails that we found worthy of noting.

In addition to the two routes we covered in **New Haven**, another place to run or walk is **Edgewood Park**. This area, near the Yale Bowl, is very pretty and you can run through some great neighborhoods with many older ornate homes. Our only reservation with Edgewood Park is that, despite being only two miles from downtown New Haven, you really need to drive and park there. We tried to get there on foot from downtown, but found ourselves in some very poor and unattractive suburbs. While we saw no major safety threats, it is not something we could recommend.

New London, another major Connecticut city, is home of the U.S. Coast Guard Academy[4] and the Naval Submarine Base New London.[5] Apart from its military facilities, New London is not a big travel destination and is predominantly an industrial city. It has a new waterfront park downtown, but no on-foot trails *per se*. For on-foot exercise, we explored the vicinity of **Ocean Beach**, the best nearby beach. We found the occasional jogger around here, but failed in pinning down any route that meets our criteria. Also in New London, the **Arboretum of Connecticut College** has a popular trail system.[6]

---

2   See: www.greenwichct.org/ParksAndRec/prFABrucePark.pdf
3   See: http://www.railtrails.org/newsandpubs/trailofthemonth/archives/0604.html
4   See: www.cga.edu
5   See: www.subasenlon.navy.mil
6   See: www.conncoll.edu

Shelton is between Bridgeport and Waterbury, off Route 8. It has a lovely trail system in what is known as the Shelton Lakes Greenway, including a 4.5-mile main recreation path.[7]

In **Stamford**, our first route touched on the Mill River, the name applied to the lower eight miles of the Rippowam River as it passes through the city to Long Island Sound. There are plans to further improve this area and build **Mill River Park**. Watch for major inner-city on-foot trails resulting from that development.

Also in Stamford, there are on-foot trails at the 63-acre **Bartlett Arboretum**, about six miles north of downtown. About four miles northwest of downtown Stamford, on the Stamford-Greenwich line, there is another network of trails in **Mianus River Park**. It can be reached from a trailhead in Merriebrook Lane in Stamford or a trailhead on Cognewaugh Road in Greenwich.

In **Stratford**, east of Bridgeport, there is some excellent coastal running in the Lordship area. On this quiet peninsula, south of the Bridgeport Municipal Airport, there are stretches of road right along the Sound—something that is not particularly common in Connecticut.

Waterbury is one of the state's largest cities, and most New Englanders know the main highway through it well. However, I drew a blank in trying to find interesting on-foot routes in this city. I look forward to hearing from Waterbury residents willing to share their own secret ideas.

Connecticut also has some interesting rail-trails which are not convenient to cities. However, for a place to drive to and jog, these are interesting possibilities. For more details, see *The Official Rails-to-Trails Conservancy Guidebook.*[8]

* * * *

Connecticut has many pleasant places to get out on-foot, especially in its small communities. The cities are not the high points of this state. We have described what we believe are the best on-foot routes convenient to cities, and leave it to you to discover the rest.

Incidentally, for serious Connecticut runners, we recommend the website www.hitekracing.com.

---

7   See: www.sheltontrails.org
8   By Cynthia Mascott, 2000, published by The Globe Pequot Press.

Pine Tree State: Maine

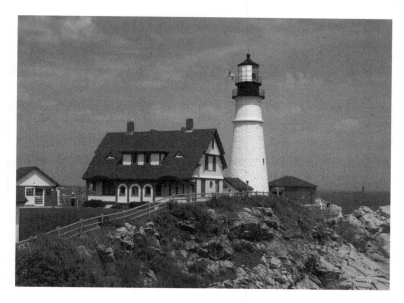

Maine was part of Massachusetts until 1820, when it was spun off and joined the Union as the 23rd state. It is well known today for its rugged and scenic coastline, lighthouses, countless lakes, forests, and summer and winter resorts.

Maine has the third-largest population of the New England states, despite being the most geographically remote. Maine's population, however, is widely distributed over the state's area, with relatively few major concentrations of residents.

In fact, there is only one city center with a population exceeding 50,000 inhabitants—Greater Portland, the business capital of the state, with a regional population of around 230,000. Therefore, this chapter focuses most on Greater Portland. The other center of special significance to visitors is the state capital, Augusta, which we made sure to cover fully. There are many good on-foot routes around other Maine cities and towns as well, as noted in the Other Routes section.

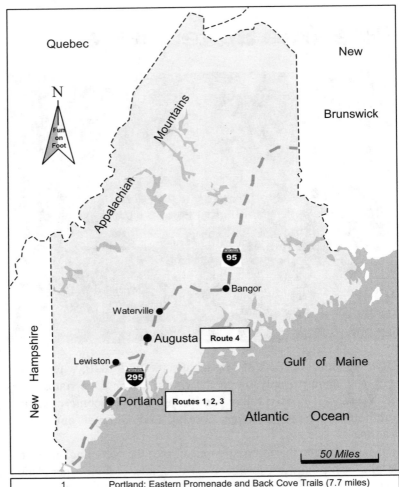

1.	Portland: Eastern Promenade and Back Cove Trails (7.7 miles)	
2.	Portland: Peaks Island (4.0 miles)	
3.	Portland-South Portland: Harborwalk and Greenbelt (8.1 miles)	
4.	Augusta: Greenway and Arboretum (4.9 miles)	

Maine Featured Routes

Portland: Eastern Promenade and Back Cove Trails

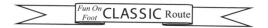

Distance	7.7 miles
Comfort	There is no more comfortable trail anywhere! This route follows marked well-maintained multi-use trails all the way. The trail surfaces are mostly paved, with some gravel parts. In the summer, there are ample restroom and water-fountain facilities. Expect plenty of other people sharing the trail, including many joggers. The Eastern Promenade Trail is good for inline skating but not the Back Cove Trail.
Attractions	The scenic beauty of Portland Harbor and Back Cove, and the company of so many friendly Maine outdoor-lovers, make this trail outstandingly attractive. Passing by the narrow gauge railway system adds an interesting element.
Convenience	Start and finish in the Old Port area of downtown Portland, close to the ferry terminal, the business district, the main tourist hotels, and attractions.
Destination	Pick your own favorite destination spot in Portland's Old Port area. If interested in food or beverage, there are many excellent restaurants and pubs here, including places on the harbor shore.

Portland, first settled by the British in 1632, is a city with enormous character. It has been primarily a shipping port since the American Revolution. The Old Port area has been recently rejuvenated into a lively and popular tourist area, complete with cobblestone streets, appealing shops, and some excellent restaurants and pubs.

Outdoor exercise is high on the city's agenda and, thanks largely to the efforts of the outstanding Portland Trails organization, there are some well-marked and well-maintained pedestrian trails.[1] This route combines two trails supported by that organization.

---

1   The Portland Trails non-profit organization; see: http://www.trails.org

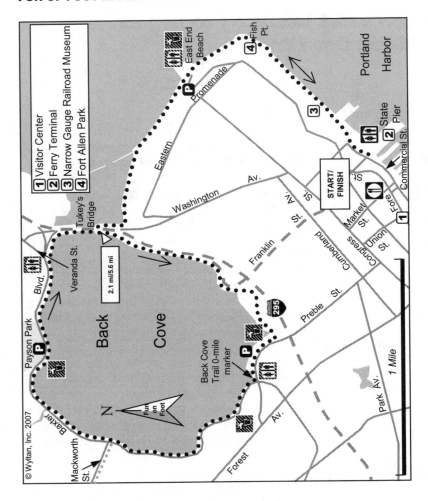

Start at the Maine State Pier, which is on Commercial Street at the lower end of Franklin Street. Pick up the shared-use trail heading east. Pass the narrow gauge railway terminal and museum. There are views of Fort Gorges in Casco Bay. Continue through Fort Allen Park and on to East End Beach, a popular local beach. After passing the water treatment plant you come to Tukey's Bridge, the bridge carrying Interstate 295. Follow the trail around under the bridge and up to where it meets the Back Cove Trail.

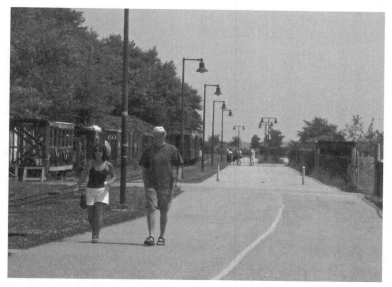

Eastern Promenade Trail, Narrow Gauge Railroad on Left

One thing that struck us about running on Portland's trails is the friendliness of the people. Everyone exchanges greetings—this is so different from Boston!

Back Cove is 3.5 miles around and the trail has half-mile markers. The 0-mile reference is where Preble Street Extension intersects Baxter Boulevard (about 1.5 miles clockwise from Tukey's Bridge). You can go around the loop either way—we arbitrarily chose to go clockwise.

The first mile tracks the Interstate, but is far enough away to be pleasant. Then the trail leaves the highway and follows the shore with only quiet streets nearby. There are more than enough water fountains and portable restrooms along the way in the summer season.

VARIATION

You can follow Mackworth Street on the west side of the loop to connect with Baxter Woods, a 30-acre wooded nature preserve, and the University of New England campus.

Complete the loop around to Tukey's Bridge. Cross the bridge on the west-side walkway, back to the point where you joined the loop

---

from the Eastern Promenade. Retrace your outbound route on the Eastern Promenade Trail back to the Old Port area.

If you need a snack or beverage break after your outing, there is no shortage of great places in either Commercial Street or a short block north in Fore Street, around Market Street. Every time Nola and I have visited Portland, we have had a blast! We can personally recommend the Old Port Tavern, Gritty McDuff's, Bull Feeney's, the Ri Ra Irish Pub, and the Dry Dock.

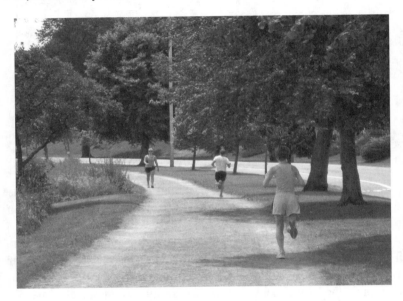

Back Cove Trail is Joggers' Paradise

Portland: Peaks Island

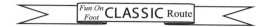

Distance	4.0 miles
Comfort	The entire route is along street sidewalks or edges, but there is little traffic and vehicles move slowly. On a nice day expect plenty of other pedestrians and cyclists on the same route. Not recommended for inline skating.
Attractions	Beautiful scenic views of the ocean, beaches, rocks, and distant lighthouses.
Convenience	Catch a ferry service in the Old Port area of downtown Portland, close to the business district, the main tourist hotels, and attractions.
Destination	There are some excellent food and beverage places near the island's ferry terminal, where you can relax waiting for the next ferry to the mainland.

If you have half a day to spare in Portland, this is an excellent way to spend it. Catch the Casco Bay Lines ferry to Peaks Island from the Maine State Pier, on Commercial Street at the lower end of Franklin Street. There are several ferries per day and the ride, which takes about 20 minutes, is particularly scenic and enjoyable. On the island, do a four-mile loop that hugs the coastline for much of the way. This route has also been recommended by the Portland Trails organization.

The outbound ferry delivers you to Forest City Landing at the end of Welch Street. Virtually all of the island's commercial establishments are clustered around here. Go up Welch Street and turn right into the main street, Island Avenue. Follow that street until it swings left and changes name to New Island Avenue. Take the second right into Whitehead Street, which leads you into Seashore Avenue, the main road around the south and west coasts of the island.

The road around the island is very pleasant, with quite a few beautiful homes on the left and sea views on the right. Since there is no sidewalk for much of the way, you often have to use the edge of the road. However, this is not a cause for concern. We found plenty of other pedestrians doing this route, along with many cyclists. The few

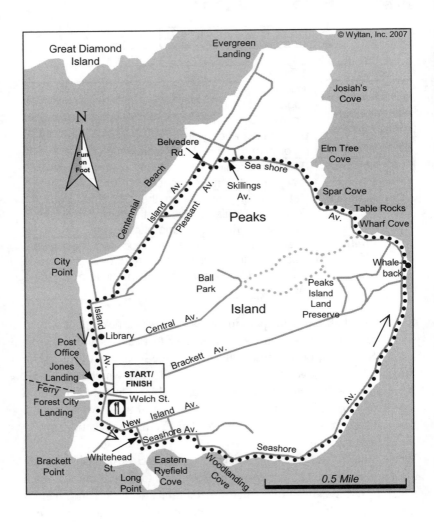

© Wyltan, Inc. 2007

vehicles encountered travel slowly and drivers are relaxed and patient. The people you meet are universally smiling and friendly. You could not find a more enjoyable on-foot outing anywhere.

Follow the road around to the unmistakable rock formation called Whaleback, a popular fishing spot.

VARIATION

There are some footpaths across the island a little north of Whaleback. These paths go through a conservation area and then connect with Central Avenue, which leads back to Island Avenue close to the commercial area and ferry terminal. You can cut through here if you wish.

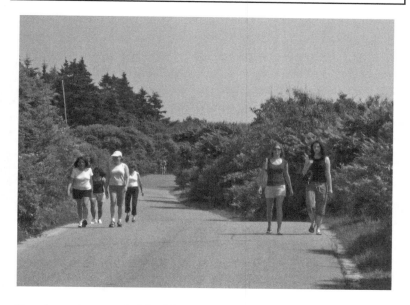

Seashore Avenue is Used by Pedestrians as Much as Vehicles

Seashore Avenue continues past Wharf Cove and Spar Cove and the adjacent rocky shore. Then the road heads inland. Continue to where Seashore Avenue swings right and Skillings Avenue bears off to the left. Skillings Avenue leads to Pleasant Avenue. Go left into Pleasant Avenue and then take the first right, Belvedere Road, to Island Avenue. Take Island Avenue south, all the way back to the commercial area.

The only deficiency we found in this route was an absence of restrooms and water along the way. Be sure to carry water. There are restrooms at the ferry terminal and, when it is open, the library in Island Avenue.

When you finish the loop, you might welcome the opportunity for a food and beverage stop before catching a return ferry. The places we can recommend are all on Island Avenue: The Pub at the Inn at Welch

Street; the Cockeyed Gull a block north; and Peak Island House a block south.

We had no hesitation in making this route a Fun-on-Foot Classic. The on-foot conditions, beautiful homes, scenic beauty, and friendly people add up to make this a route that no one should miss.

Portland-South Portland: Harborwalk and Greenbelt

Distance	8.1 miles
Comfort	Follow street sidewalks for 4.4 miles, and a well-maintained paved pedestrian and bicycle trail for 3.7 miles. Expect plenty of other pedestrians around. Mostly suitable for inline skating.
Attractions	See the Portland Harbor from many different aspects, including an exhilarating view while crossing the Casco Bay Bridge. Follow the pleasant and popular South Portland Greenbelt Walkway. Go through several parks in South Portland, including Bug Light Park where you see the cute Bug Light at first hand and where locals fly their kites. You can also see the Portland Harbor Museum and Fort Preble. This is an out-and-back route but, subject to bus schedules, you can take a bus one-way and halve the distance.
Convenience	Start and finish in the Old Port area of downtown Portland, close to the ferry terminal, the business district, the main tourist hotels, and attractions.
Destination	Pick your own favorite destination spot in Portland's Old Port area. If interested in food or beverage, there are many excellent restaurants and pubs here, including places on the harbor shore.

We try to avoid out-and-back routes but this one has so much going for it we would be remiss in omitting it. You get to exercise in an excellent environment on the South Portland Greenbelt and also enjoy the many views of the Portland Harbor. In fact, you can even avoid the out-and-back characteristic on all days except Sundays, by using a bus for either the outbound or return.

Start at the Maine State Pier, on Commercial Street at the lower end of Franklin Street. Follow the Harborwalk trail signs south down Commercial Street. At some stage, such as at High Street, cross to the west side, that is the inland side, of Commercial Street. Keep following the trail signs going under the Casco Bay Bridge and then looping back up to York Street. The signs then lead you across two streets, and eventually to the east-side walkway of the bridge.

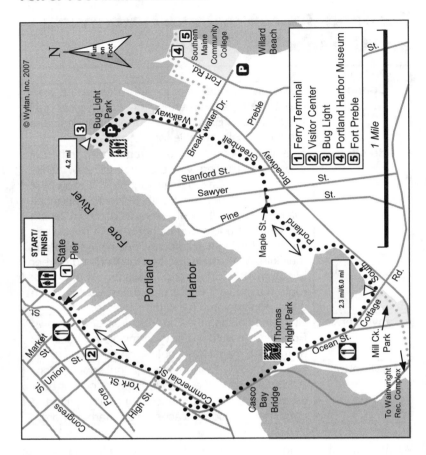

VARIATION

There is an easier way onto the bridge, which saves you 0.2 miles and the street crossings. Simply follow High Street up to York Street and turn left, leading directly to the bridge walkway. In our mileage for this route, we have assumed you will follow that route on the return leg.

The Casco Bay Bridge crossing is excellent for on-footers. The walkway is dedicated to pedestrians—bikes must use the road—and the view is nothing short of spectacular. After crossing the water, but long before the end of the bridge, there is a pedestrian ramp down to the left.

Uncharacteristically for Portland, there is no sign. However, be sure to take this ramp down to Thomas Knight Park, under the bridge approach on the South Portland side. There is a seasonal water fountain here.

Follow the sidewalk of Ocean Street, noting the bars and restaurants here that you might want to drop into on your return trip. At the major road branch, bear left following the sidewalk of Cottage Road through the shopping area. This takes you to Mill Creek Park, and the intersection with the South Portland Greenbelt Walkway.

The Greenbelt Walkway is a paved rail-trail, stretching from the Wainwright Recreation Complex in the south, through Mill Creek Park, to Bug Light Park. It is equally popular with local joggers, cyclists, and strolling families.

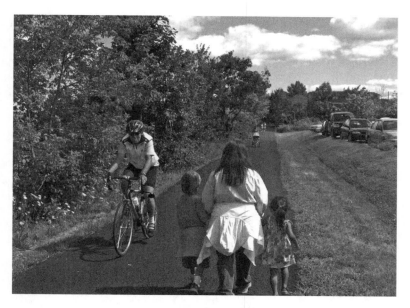

The South Portland Greenbelt Walkway

The trail is simple to follow. Just note that when you get to Pine Street (at the Ferry Village sign), you need to follow the sidewalk of Maple Street to Sawyer Street.

At Breakwater Drive, the trail splits and you face a decision. The left branch takes you to Bug Light Park. The Bug Light is the small but classy light signaling the entrance to Portland Harbor. Bug Light Park is also a popular place for kite flying and boat launching. There are seasonal restrooms here.

If you follow the southerly trail option at Breakwater Drive, you come to the small Portland Harbor Museum, Fort Preble (with an active history spanning 1808 to 1950), and the campus of the South Maine Community College.

If you want to use a bus for either the outbound or return Portland trip, there is a direct bus service operated by the City of South Portland Bus Service to Willard Square and the Southern Maine Community College. When we were last there, there was a half-hour service on weekdays, a less frequent service on Saturdays, and no service at all on Sundays. Hopefully, they will correct the latter eccentricity some time soon.

If you plan to follow our basic route recommendation and return back to Portland via the Greenbelt and Harborwalk, remember there are several places to stop for a drink or snack in South Portland between Mill Creek and the Casco Bay Bridge, should you need a break. Otherwise, just continue back to Old Port and have fun there!

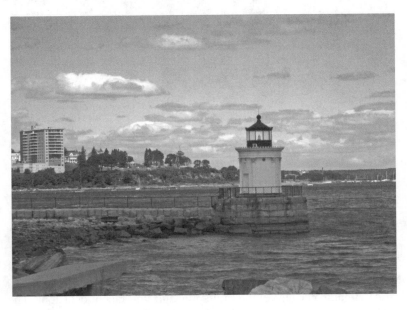

The Bug Light at Portland Harbor's Entrance

Augusta: Greenway and Arboretum

Distance	4.9 miles
Comfort	Most of this route is on off-road, well-maintained trails. Some parts are paved and others are unpaved. The going is mostly level. Expect plenty of other people around, mostly relaxed locals, but no crowds. The riverside sections are suitable for inline skating, but not the arboretum trails.
Attractions	The natural beauty of the trail system along the Kennebec River, the historic sites of Old Fort Western and the Kennebec Arsenal, and the interesting and varied terrain and plant life of the Pine Tree State Arboretum.
Convenience	Start and end near the post office in Water Street, in the center of Augusta. Alternatively, start and/or finish at the State Capitol, about a mile from the post office via a multi-use trail. If staying in a hotel on Interstate 95, it is about two miles to the post office, and we suggest you drive that distance and park nearby.
Destination	The center of Augusta, with such attractions as the State Capitol and the Maine State Museum. There are also local restaurants and bars.

Maine's first state capital, from 1820 to 1832, was Portland. Augusta, considered more centrally located, became the capital in 1832.

Augusta is a small, quiet city with a population under 20,000. The city's heart, on the Kennebec River, is very peaceful—most of the shopping malls, hotels, and nightlife establishments are about two miles away, clustered around two Interstate-95 interchanges.

However, if you are seeking great outdoor exercise places, look to the trails near the river. If necessary, drive here from the Interstate, since the roads in are not particularly pedestrian-friendly.

There are three popular running-place choices: the Augusta Greenway, mainly on the east bank of the river; the Pine Tree State Arboretum, also on the east side of the river; and the Kennebec River Rail Trail along the west bank of the river. We decided to craft a nice route from the city center that incorporates the first two options. We shall also discuss how to link in the third option.

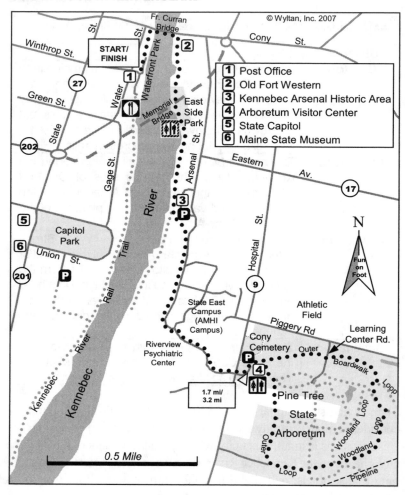

We assume a start near the central post office, on Water Street at Winthrop Street.

VARIATION

If you want to start from or finish near the State Capitol, there is an excellent way to get to or from the post office on foot. You can access the Kennebec River Rail Trail near the post office. You can also access it from the trailhead near the parking area off Union Street near Capitol Park. Using this path adds about a mile each way to our route mileage.

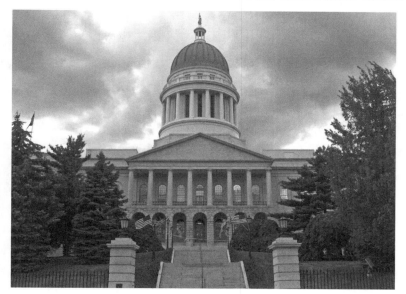

The Maine State Capitol

From the river end of Winthrop Street, follow the trail north up the river through Waterfront Park. Cross the Father Curran Bridge, and go immediately right onto the start of the Augusta Greenway Trail. Pass Old Fort Western on your left.

Continue to Eastside Park, which has a playground and restrooms. You then come to the Kennebec Arsenal Historic Area. Pass the old arsenal buildings and proceed to the parking lot. Climb the hill heading away from the river and pick up the sidewalk of Arsenal Street, continuing in the same southerly direction. Pass the big smokestack on your left, the gazebo, and then the gray stone buildings that headquartered the historic 1840-vintage, but now defunct, Augusta Mental Health Institute (AMHI).

Arsenal Street then swings to the left away from the river. Keep following it and the signs to Hospital Street. Where you meet Hospital Street, cross the road and enter the Pine Tree State Arboretum. Try to pick up an Arboretum trail map from either the visitor center or from a box at the trailhead at the north end of the parking lot.[2]

---

2   A map is available from the website: http://www. pinetreestatearboretum.org

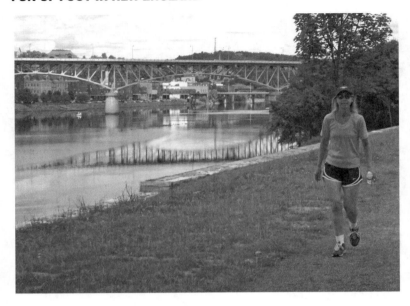

The Augusta Greenway

It is not an enormous arboretum, but a very pleasant one from the outdoor exerciser's perspective. There are lots of trails and you will generally find many other joggers around here, in addition to plant enthusiasts.

The simplest approach for the jogger is to take the Outer Loop, which is quite well signposted. The only possible problem is that the southeastern piece of that loop can become somewhat muddy if there has been recent rain, so you would be safer to pick up the southern and western segments of the Woodland Loop (as per our map) instead. The Woodland Loop is particularly pleasant, passing through a heavy growth forest. The northern part of the Outer Loop involves a boardwalk across some wetlands terrain, where there is interesting wildlife. Cross the access road called Learning Center Road, and continue on the Outer Loop back to the Arboretum car park. Retrace your footsteps from there back to the center of Augusta.

If you want to stop for a food or beverage break in Augusta after that little exercise outing, there are not a lot of choices. We can definitely recommend Delia's Irish Pub at 349 Water Street, close to the end of our nominal route. This seemed to us the most fully rounded pub-restaurant in the central city area. It has good food, is popular, and has all the usual Irish pub appeal.

Other Routes

The largest population center of Maine is **Greater Portland**, including the cities/towns of **Portland**, **South Portland**, **Falmouth** and **Cape Elizabeth**. We earlier featured three routes, convenient to downtown Portland. Here are some ideas for other routes in the region... [3]

North of Portland there is a very pleasant 1.25-mile walk or run around **Mackworth Island**, plus some short side-trails. You can run from downtown Portland via the sidewalks of Veranda Street (reachable from the north end of the Tukey's Bridge walkway), Route 1, and Andrews Avenue. However, this is not an enormously pleasant on-foot route so the more common approach is to drive to the island's parking lot off Route 1 and do the route from there.

In **South Portland**, the Greenbelt Walkway that we introduced earlier also connects from where we joined it (at Mill Creek Park) to the Wainwright Recreation Complex in the southwesterly direction.

There are some very pleasant short walks around **Fort Williams** and the **Portland Head Light**, the signature Maine lighthouse, pictured at the chapter head. This site is in the town of Cape Elizabeth. While it is certainly possible to run here and back from the Willard Beach area or anywhere else in South Portland, the routes involve quite ordinary, uninspiring street sidewalks.

The **Fore River Sanctuary**, west of downtown Portland but east of Interstate 95, is an 85-acre wildlife sanctuary with two miles of pedestrian trails. A trail to here up the Fore River from downtown Portland is partly complete.

* * * *

Outside the Greater Portland area, here are some other notable on-foot routes in Maine...

Scenic **Acadia National Park**, near the town of **Bar Harbor** on **Mount Desert Island**, has an extensive network of historic carriage roads, on which pedestrians mostly have free rein. The park also has other hiking trails and a limited number of vehicle roads. The options here are too extensive for us to present any simple formula. If you get to this park, stop by the Hulls Cove Visitor Center or the Park Headquarters to pick up a map and further information, allowing you

---

3   For more ideas, see http://www.trails.org

to plan your on-foot outings. Limited information is available on-line.[4]
There is also a short, but scenic, Shore Path along the coast south from
Bar Harbor.

In **Bangor** there are several miles of trails in 650-acre Bangor City
Forest, north of the city center.[5]

In **Bethel** there is a new multi-use trail from Davis Park on Route 2
East (Main Street) a little less than a mile along the Androscoggin River
to Route 2 West (Mayville Road). If staying in town, you can build
this into a comfortable jogging loop. Looking ahead, an active trails
committee is working to expand the present trail in both directions to
give several miles of trails, including a link to the public high school's
track facility.[6]

Around **Boothbay Harbor** there are over 25 miles of hiking trails
on various publicly accessible properties. Maps and directions are
available from the Boothbay Region Land Trust.[7]

In **Brunswick** there is a 2.6-mile paved multi-use path called the
Androscoggin River Bicycle and Pedestrian Path, which is popular
with local joggers.[8]

Camden is a seaside town on the edge of Camden Hills State Park.[9]
You can hike from the town up 780-foot Mount Battie for some excellent
views. Beyond Mount Battie there are 30 more miles of hiking trails,
including a trail to the top of 1,385-foot Mount Megunticook.

At **Carrabassett Valley**, near Sugarloaf Mountain, there is a popular 5.5-mile rural multi-use trail called the Narrow Gauge Pathway.[10]

There is a 15-mile gravel multi-use trail between **Farmington** and
Jay, but I understand it is quite rugged and more suited to hiking and
off-road vehicle use than running or jogging.

We mentioned the **Kennebec River Rail Trail** in our Augusta route
description. When complete (expected soon), this trail will extend from
Augusta 6.5 miles south to the towns of **Hallowell** and **Gardiner**.

In **Lewiston/Auburn**, there are some mapped-out on-foot loops
with lengths of one to four miles. I cannot speak authoritatively as to

4   See: http://www.nps.gov/acad/index.htm
5   See: http://www.bangormaine.gov/vb_recreation.php
6   See: http://www.bethelmaine.com/recreation-activities/summer
7   See: http://www.bbrlt.org/Hiking.htm
8   See: http://www.brunswickme.org/parkrec/androscogginriverbp.htm
9   See: http://www.state.me.us/doc/parks/index.html
10   See: http://www.carrabassettvalley.org/attractions/Narrowgauge.asp

their quality. Summaries and a map are available from the Androscoggin Transportation Resource Center.[11]

At **Ogonquit** there is a popular 1.5-mile scenic coastal trail, the **Marginal Way**, heading south to Perkins Cove. Start from either end, and run or walk the trail out-and-back. There are snack places at both ends and good wind-down pub-restaurants in Ogonquit.

At **Orono**, north of Bangor, the University of Maine has an extensive trail system on University-owned land adjacent to the campus. There is also a paved bike path from the campus to the center of the City of Old Town. A map is available from the University website.[12]

Waterville and its neighboring towns of **Winslow**, **Fairfield**, **Benton**, and **Oakland** have some excellent trails and a very active trails advocacy group.[13] There is a trail network at Colby College, handy to downtown Waterville on its west side. About two miles north of downtown, there is the 1.8-mile Benton-Winslow Rotary Centennial Trail. This is a well-maintained rail trail along the Kennebec River into Fairfield, ideal for running. About a mile northwest of downtown Waterville is a new 1.5-mile trail along Messalonskee Stream. Other trail segments exist, and further pieces are being progressively built, filling in a planned network of 24 miles of trail along the Kennebec River and Messalonskee Stream.

York has some particularly picturesque oceanside trails. The **Fisherman's Walk** connects York Harbor with York Village (also known as Old York). The **Cliff Walk** is a very attractive path which starts at the end of York Harbor Beach and weaves along the cliffs between the ocean and historic homes and cottages.

For further ideas for on-foot routes in Maine, check out the website of the Healthy Maine Walks organization.[14]

---

11   See: http://www.atrcmpo.org
12   See: http://www.umaine.edu/campusrecreation/trails.asp
13   See: http://www.kmtrails.org
14   See: http://www.healthymainewalks.org

8

Granite State: New Hampshire

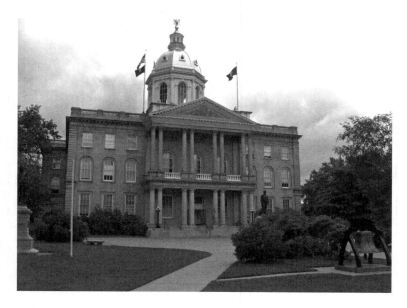

The ninth state, New Hampshire, is notable for its variety of environments. It has New England's most spectacular mountain terrain, including such hiker-popular peaks as Mount Washington and Mount Monadnock. It has some beautiful lake regions. It has only a tiny piece of coastline, sandwiched between the Massachusetts and Maine shores, but the scenic beauty of that piece of coast is second to none. Meanwhile, its largest population areas in the south of the state mostly have industrial backgrounds.

Running, jogging, and walking are popular activities throughout the state. Many centers and regions have trail systems. You will feel

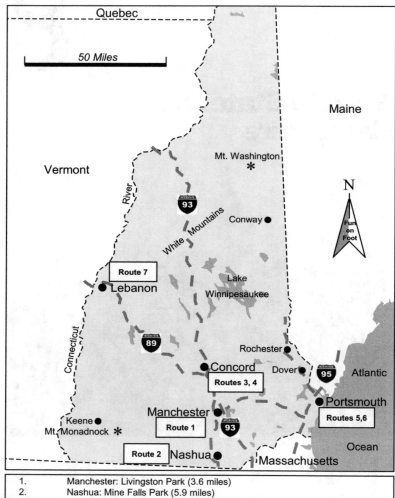

1.	Manchester: Livingston Park (3.6 miles)
2.	Nashua: Mine Falls Park (5.9 miles)
3.	Concord: City Connection to Seekamp Trail (4.1 miles)
4.	Concord: Merrill Park and SPNHF Trails (6.1 miles)
5.	Portsmouth: Peirce Island (2.6 miles)
6.	Portsmouth: New Castle Loop (6.9 miles)
7.	Lebanon: Northern Rail Trail and Mill Road (7.7 miles)

New Hampshire Featured Routes

comfortable being out on foot almost anywhere in this state. Even the more industrial cities have comparatively low crime rates.

There are several sizable cities in New Hampshire, but no major metropolitan areas *per se*. The only cities with populations over 40,000 are Manchester, Nashua, and Concord. We made sure to cover on-foot routes in these centers. Of the smaller cities, the most interesting one is unquestionably Portsmouth, a popular tourist destination on the coast, with a fascinating history and great scenery. We feature two excellent routes there. The other city we cover is Lebanon, located at the intersection of the Interstate 91 and 89 highway systems and the main gateway point between New Hampshire and Vermont.

Manchester: Livingston Park

Distance	3.6 miles
Comfort	Use street sidewalks 1.1 miles each way between downtown and Livingston Park. Do 1.4 miles (or more by running circuits) inside park on excellent pedestrian trails. The street sidewalks are through respectable neighborhoods with people around, and you can avoid heavily trafficked streets. Inside the park, expect plenty of other people, including runners, joggers, and walkers. Not suitable for inline skating.
Attractions	Livingston Park is an attractive park with leafy trails around a pleasant lake. There is also a professional quality athletic track where you can run quarter-mile circuits.
Convenience	Start and finish in downtown Manchester, close to hotels and local businesses.
Destination	Downtown Manchester, with numerous good pubs, restaurants, and shops.

Manchester, with a population of a little over 100,000, is New Hampshire's largest city. The best on-foot exercise place near downtown Manchester is Livingston Park, a little over a mile from the center of downtown. You can drive and park there and then exercise, but we have included in our route the on-foot travel from and to downtown.

We nominally start at City Hall at the intersection of Elm Street and Hanover Street. There are many choices of routes to the park, through Manchester's neat rectangular street grid. We suggest you use one of the quieter streets, such as Walnut Street, for the north-south part of the route. Go east on Hanover Street to the little park where Walnut Street starts, and follow Walnut Street up to Webster Street. Cross Webster Street, go one short block east, and turn left into busy Hooksett Road (Routes 3 and 28).

Go up Hooksett Road about a hundred yards to the Livingston Park entrance on your left. Follow the path to the athletic field.

You have a couple of choices as to how to exercise on foot in this park. If you are a serious athlete, there is a professional quality running track around the athletic field, which is very popular with fitness-conscious locals. The inside lane is exactly a quarter-mile.   Do as

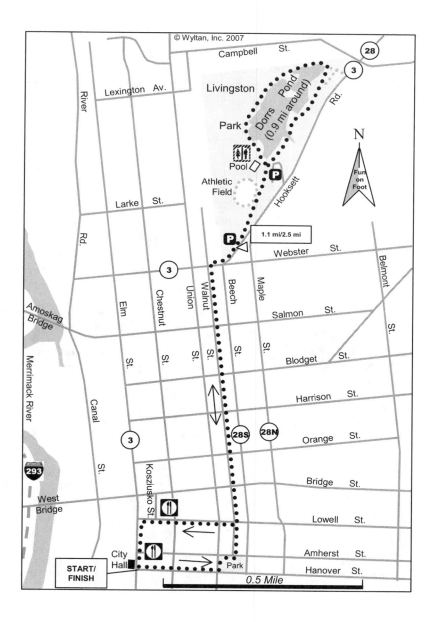

© Wyltan, Inc. 2007

many circuits as you wish. Another option is a 0.9-mile nature trail around Dorrs Pond. For our featured route we chose to include a loop of the latter.

From the athletic field, go north past the parking lots and playground to the nature trail trailhead. Go around the lake, enjoying the pleasant, shady conditions in the forest surroundings. The trail is gravel and excellent for running or walking as you prefer. Expect many other pedestrians sharing the trail.

If the pool at the south end of the pond is open, you can use the restrooms here.

When finished with Livingston Park, retrace your steps to downtown. If you are ready for a food and beverage break, I suggest following Lowell Street back to the Elm Street vicinity. There are two excellent Irish Pubs that Nola and I have particularly enjoyed. The first is the Wild Rover Pub in Kosziusko Street, near Lowell and Elm. We found good food and excellent service there. Another good Irish Pub is the beautifully decorated Shaskeen in Elm Street just north of Hanover Street.

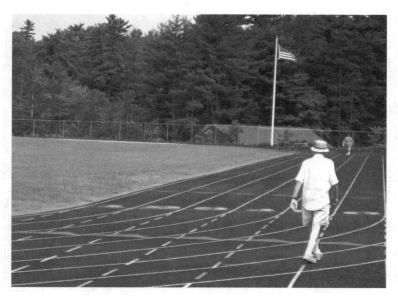

Livingston Park Athletic Field Track

Nashua: Mine Falls Park

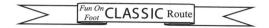

Distance	5.9 miles
Comfort	It is a half-mile each way between Main Street and the start of the park trail system, via good street sidewalks. The 4.9 miles of park trails have varied surfaces, mostly well-maintained unpaved trails. Some trails are paved. Some parts are narrow and have moderate grades, but most athletically inclined people can easily run the entire route. Expect to pass other pedestrians but do not expect crowds. Not suitable for inline skating.
Attractions	A very pleasant escape into a wilderness setting, close to the center of the city. The mill pond and canal system is interesting to observe.
Convenience	Start and finish on Main Street at the river bridge, in the center of Nashua.
Destination	Downtown Nashua, with pubs, restaurants, and a range of shops.

Nashua is New Hampshire's second-largest city, with a population around 90,000. The city proudly boasts that it is the only city in the nation to twice win *Money* magazine's award for "Best Place to Live in America."

One reason why Nashua is a great place to live is unquestionably its city park system. The most prominent park is 325-acre Mine Falls Park, in the middle of the city. Mine Falls Park occupies the undeveloped land around the Nashua River and the canal system that powered the mills of the Nashua Manufacturing Company for many years.

According to Nashua City, the name Mine Falls derives from lead mining near the falls at the park's southwest end in the 1700s. The park lies between the Nashua River and the canal for the roughly 3-mile stretch from the dam and falls to the Millyard area, where the Nashua Manufacturing Company once operated. The canal carried water from above the falls to power the mills with a 36-foot head of water.

The park has several defined trails, marked with colored-diamond blazes. Unfortunately, the blazes are often hard to see. Also, good

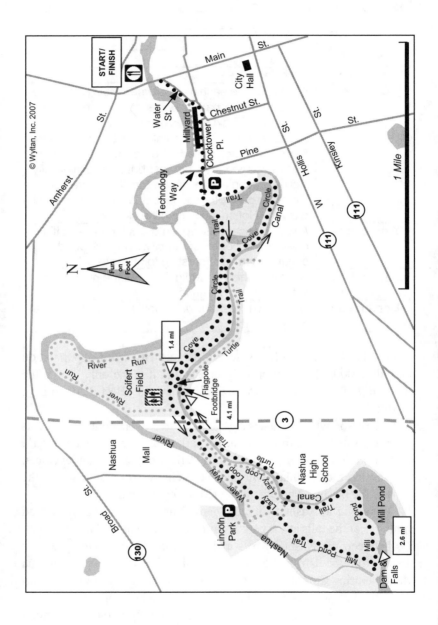

maps are not easy to find. When I last checked, the map available on the city's website was quite rudimentary.[1] We did pick up a paper map from the Nashua Parks and Recreation Department's office, but finding that office is too much trouble for the average visitor. Accordingly, we have tried to show the essential aspects of the trail system on our map.

The main marked trails are:[2]

> Mill Pond Trail (1.26 miles): Orange blaze;
> Turtle Trail (1.58 miles paved): Purple blaze;
> River Run Trail (1.35 miles): Yellow blaze;
> Cove Circle Trail (2.23 miles): Green blaze;
> Lazy Loop Trail (about 1.4 miles): Blue blaze;
> Water Way Trail (about 0.3 miles): Red blaze.

For our nominal route, we chose a basic loop from the park entry point nearest Main Street to the dam and falls, returning a different way. The route uses the Cove Circle, Lazy Loop, Mill Pond, and Turtle Trails, and you can optionally tack on a loop of the River Run Trail.

When Nola and I did this loop, we encountered quite a few runners, walkers, and cyclists, including females alone. However, some parts are secluded so you might prefer to go with a companion.

We assume a start in downtown Nashua, where Main Street crosses the Nashua River. Follow the river on its south side towards the west, using pedestrian paths and sidewalks along Water Street. Go through the industrial area that is now designated the Nashua Manufacturing Company Historic District and is more commonly called the Millyard. When we were there, you had a choice of ways through it. You can go through the rear parking area of the old mill buildings, which is not a bad choice since it follows the river and there is virtually no traffic. Alternatively, on the other side of the mill buildings is Clocktower Place, which you can follow to its end. In either case, you come to a commercial and light industrial area. Go in the general direction that is a straight extension of Clocktower Place, passing the sign to Technology Way off to the right.

Suddenly you come upon a trailhead to Mine Falls Park, exiting directly from the light industrial area. This is known as the Pine Street access to Mine Falls Park.

---

1   See: http://www.gonashua.com
2   Mileages are taken from the Nashua Parks and Recreation Department's map.

Take the north branch of the Cove Circle Trail along the river. This trail is mostly through woods and is shady and quiet. Unfortunately, the green markers for this trail are rarely visible within the surrounding greenery. The trail takes you to a major trail junction where there is a flagpole, and a path to a footbridge over the canal to your left. Go straight ahead, keeping the canal to your left. There are seasonal restrooms to your right at the sporting fields.

VARIATION

At this point, you can add in a 1.35-mile loop of the River Run Trail if you wish. This trail hugs the bank of the Nashua River and circumnavigates the sporting fields area.

Continue west to the underpass under the major highway, Route 3. After the highway, the trail forks. I suggest keeping to the right, which leads to the northern branch of the Lazy Loop Trail and the nearby Water Way Trail. Follow either of these.

Cross a paved trail, the western end of Turtle Trail. Following the paved trail to the right would take you across the river to Lincoln Park, another primary access point to Mine Falls Park. For our route, however, go essentially straight ahead into the western branch of the Mill Pond Trail.

Cross the footbridge over the babbling brook and continue on to the dam and the falls. This is a beautiful spot to take a short break.

From the dam and falls, go back into Mine Falls Park, bear right, and follow the branch of the Mill Pond Trail around the Mill Pond. This trail is very pleasant and shady and follows the northern bank of the canal after the Mill Pond.

You again meet the paved trail, Turtle Trail, at its bridge across the canal. Cross the bridge to the rear of the high school, and take advantage of the nicely paved Turtle Trail up the south bank of the canal. On reaching the next footbridge, you can see the flagpole across the canal and recognize that you were here on your outbound journey.

Cross the footbridge back to the north side of the canal and go immediately right onto the south branch of the Cove Circle Trail. While most of our route is shady, this stretch is sunny. Nola and I were here on a 100-degrees summer day and started to struggle along this stretch.

However, the scenery along the canal is very pleasant and underfoot conditions are excellent.

This branch of the Cove Circle Trail exits into a light industrial area. Keep bearing left through the parking lots to the point at which you originally entered the park. You can use the tall Millyard smokestack to navigate back to the right general location. Retrace your original footsteps back to Main Street.

If you are interested in a food and beverage break after your outing, we found an excellent establishment here. The Peddler's Daughter is just north of the river on the east side of Main Street. It is an authentic Irish pub, but with a more innovative menu than most. I had corned beef and onions quesadillas, with salad—not really either Irish or Mexican but it sure worked for me. And the cold beer on that hot day went down extremely well.

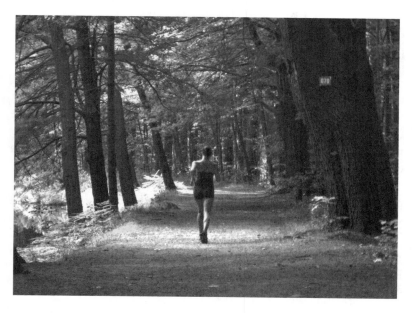

Running in Shady Mine Falls Park

Concord: City Connection to Seekamp Trail

Distance	4.1 miles
Comfort	This route involves 3.3 miles on generally good street sidewalks getting to and from the Seekamp Trail, plus a 0.8-mile loop of that trail on a good unpaved running path. Expect ample people around on all parts of the route, including runners and joggers on the Seekamp Trail. Not suitable for inline skating.
Attractions	For the runner, the main attraction is the pleasant Seekamp Trail where you should do as many loops as you wish. On the route from the city center, pass through the Concord Historic District, with several historic buildings.
Convenience	Start and finish in the center of Concord, by the State House, near city hotels.
Destination	Concord city center, with several pubs and restaurants for winding down after your outing.

Concord, New Hampshire's state capital, is the state's third-largest city, and a very pleasant, relaxed city too. For the on-foot enthusiast, the city boasts a public trails network comprising 21 trails totaling over 43 miles. Details of these trails are available from the city website,[3] and a color map and guide is available from the city information desks.

As usual, Nola and I decided to check out the quality of these trails personally. To be more precise, we chose to check out the trails that were in convenient on-foot reach of the city center. As a result, the Concord trail system gets a mixed review from us. Some of the claimed trails were in a quite sorry state and some we concluded did not even exist.[4]

3   See: http://www.onconcord.com
4   The Turkey River White Farm Trails that can be accessed from Memorial Park, 1.4 miles on foot from the city center, looked very attractive on paper. However, we found that they were badly overgrown and very unfriendly underfoot. Not surprisingly, there were no signs of people having recently used these trails at all. The East Concord Heritage Trail description mentioned a trail following West Portsmouth Street and West Locke Road. We concluded that there is no such trail, except that you can run along the edge of the road if you wish, and we would not recommend that since there is nothing interesting or attractive near there.

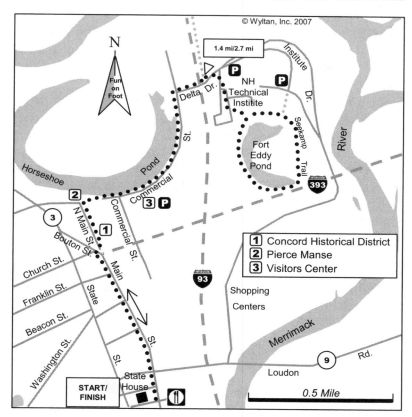

However, we found some trails northeast of the city center that were definitely worthy of featuring in this book. We present these trails in two route descriptions. This first one is good for someone seeking a place to run. The other one, in the subsequent route description, is more suited to people seeking a relaxed escape into some wilderness.

Start at the State House on Main Street at Capitol Street. Go north up Main Street, keeping to the west (left-hand) side. You come to a major intersection, where Bouton Street and the Interstate-393 connector meet Main Street. To negotiate this intersection, stay on the west side of Main Street to the pedestrian crossing across Bouton Street with the traffic signal. Cross Bouton Street here.

This brings you to a point where there is a small, quiet street, actually the extension of Main Street, leading into a picturesque area. This is the

Concord Historical District. Follow the street to its end, passing several historical houses and a plaque denoting the site of the first garrison in Concord, built in 1746, to protect against the "French and Indians." The street ends at the house that was President Pierce's Manse from 1842-48.

Turn right here following the old road (now closed to traffic) through the railroad reserve. It leads to a regular street called Commercial Street. Follow the sidewalk around the edge of Horseshoe Pond. Pass the hotel on the right and the Greater Concord Chamber of Commerce. There is a visitors center here where you can get a city map and the guide to the Concord Trail System. Continue on Commercial Street to the Delta Drive overpass across Interstate 93 to the right. Cross the overpass on its sidewalk. At the far end you find a paved bike trail heading off to the left. (We use that trail in our next route.)

For this route, go straight ahead into the campus of the New Hampshire Technical Institute. Follow the street to the right into the heart of the campus. Continue down to where you see the body of water called Fort Eddy Pond. You will here find the pedestrian trail around the pond called the Seekamp Trail. This loop of approximately 0.8 mile is popular with local runners. Our route mileage includes one loop of the Seekamp Trail but you may want to do some additional loops while here.

Retrace your original steps back to the State House. If you feel like a food and beverage break, there are several choices around the center of the city. Nola and I particularly enjoyed the Capitol Grill at Eagle Square and the Barley House, both in Main Street across from the State House.

Concord: Merrill Park and SPNHF Trails

Distance	6.1 miles
Comfort	This route involves 3.3 miles on generally good street sidewalks or quiet street edges, 1.8 miles on unpaved trails in a wilderness setting, and one mile on a paved bike path. Expect other people around on all parts of the route. Not suitable for inline skating.
Attractions	A great variety of terrain, and plant and animal life, on both the Merrill Park and SPNHF trails. On the route from the city center, pass through the Concord Historic District, with several historic buildings.
Convenience	Start and finish in the center of Concord, by the State House, near city hotels.
Destination	Concord city center, with several pubs and restaurants for winding down after your outing.

We introduced Concord and its trail system in the previous route description. This route duplicates the connection from the city center to the east side of Interstate 93 but, instead of leading to a running loop, it leads to a forest trail system more likely to excite the nature enthusiast.

Start at the State House on Main Street at Capitol Street. Go north up Main Street, keeping to the west (left-hand) side. Cross Bouton Street at the major intersection. Go through the Concord Historical District. Turn right following the old road (now closed to traffic) through the railroad reserve. Follow the sidewalk of Commercial Street around the edge of Horseshoe Pond. Continue to the Delta Drive overpass across Interstate 93 to the right. Cross the overpass on its sidewalk. At the far end you find a paved bike trail heading off to the left.

Take the paved trail for a half-mile. It crosses the Merrimack River, using the eastern edge of the Interstate-93 bridge. The trail ends in a quiet area at the intersection of Portsmouth Street and Eastman Street. There is a plaque here indicating the site of Concord's first turnpike, built in 1796. You have a couple of choices here as to the route you choose. To see the most, go straight ahead up Eastman Street, a quiet street with a sidewalk and several very old houses, some of historic sig-

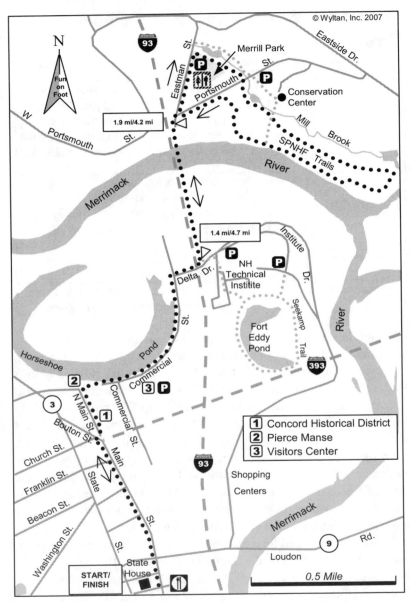

© Wyltan, Inc. 2007

N

Fun
on
Foot

I-93

Eastman St.

Merrill Park

Eastside Dr.

P

Portsmouth St.

P

Conservation
Center

W

Portsmouth St.

1.9 mi/4.2 mi

Mill Brook

SPNHF Trails

Merrimack River

1.4 mi/4.7 mi

Institute Dr.

P

NH
Technical
Institite

P

Delta Dr.

Seekamp Trail

River

Fort
Eddy
Pond

I-393

Horseshoe

Pond

Commercial St.

2

3

3

P

N Main St.

Commercial St.

3

1

Bouton St.

① Concord Historical District
② Pierce Manse
③ Visitors Center

Church St.

Main St.

I-93

Franklin St.

State

Shopping

Centers

Beacon St.

Merrimack

Washington St.

St.

9

Rd.

Loudon

START/
FINISH

State
House

0.5 Mile

nificance. You come to Merrill Park on the right. Go into the parking area. There are seasonal restrooms here, plus a playground and a pool. Go around the pool and find the trail into the woods. This is the south branch of the Merrill Park Trail, noted in the city literature. Follow the trail along the edge of Mill Brook to where it exits on Portsmouth Street.

> **VARIATION**
> You could alternatively follow the north branch of the Merrill Park Trail from Merrill Park to Portsmouth Street, although that branch is a little longer and the going is tougher. Cross the brook at the parking lot and take the trail to the right. This branch emerges on Portsmouth Street a short distance north of where the south branch emerges.

Go straight across Portsmouth Street and enter a trail that is part of the trail system known as the "Society for the Protection of New Hampshire Forests" (SPNHF) trails. Note that the main trailhead and its parking lot are a little north of here across the brook. That trailhead leads to the SPNHF Conservation Center, where you can pick up a trail map. However, when we were last here, the access from the Conservation Center to the main trails south of the brook was closed owing to flood damage, so it might be safer to just stay on the south side of the brook unless you particularly want to visit the Conservation Center.

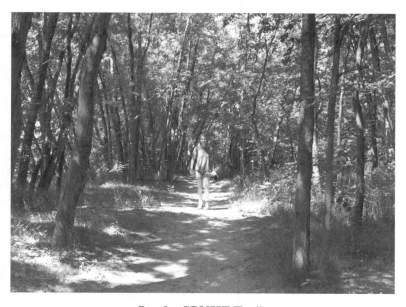

On the SPNHF Trails

Do the 1.5-mile loop of the SPNHF trails, bearing left initially, keeping the brook on your left. Continue to the riverbank, which you then follow to the right. There is an enormous variety of terrain and interesting plant and animal life in here, ranging from wetlands close to the brook, to old forests, to a nice sunny riverbank. There should be a map and guide in a trail box along the way. We found the trails to be in excellent shape, allowing running, jogging, or walking, as you prefer.

You will eventually need to take a trail to the right. This leads you back through the forest to Portsmouth Street. Follow the edge of Portsmouth Street to the left, back to the intersection with Eastman Street and the paved trail you used on your outbound leg. Retrace your original steps back to the State House.

Portsmouth: Peirce Island

Distance	2.6 miles
Comfort	This route combines 1.3 miles on one of the historic Harbor Trail walks with 0.9 mile on Peirce Island pedestrian trails and 0.4 miles on good street sidewalks connecting the two. The Harbor Trail segment may be difficult to run owing to strolling tourists, but the rest of the route is well suited to running, jogging, or walking as you choose. The route is level. Expect to encounter many other pedestrians. Not suitable for inline skating.
Attractions	Pass many historic sites, and see the various activities of Portsmouth Harbor plus Portsmouth's quaint buildings from across the water.
Convenience	Start and finish at Market Square, at the corner of Market Street (or Pleasant Street) and Congress Street in the center of Portsmouth. This is handy to city hotels and tourist attractions.
Destination	The center of Portsmouth, with innumerable historic sites plus some excellent restaurants and bars.

Portsmouth is a fascinating city. It has a history stretching back to 1623 when English settlers first moved here. It served as the state capital up until the American Revolution. It has been a major seaport, a center of industry, and a naval shipbuilding center. More recently it has been successfully converted from what was primarily an industrial city to a comfortable and popular tourist destination.

Sightseeing on foot is encouraged in Portsmouth. The local community has mapped out a set of walks, taking you past over 70 identified points of historical or other interest. If visiting, you should pay the nominal fee for a Harbor Trail map and guide available at tourist information desks. There are three walks, covering different parts of the city.

The Harbor Trail walks are not very well suited to jogging or running. However, there is one place convenient to the city with pedestrian trails suited to all forms of on-foot exercise. Peirce Island, which is connected to the city by a short causeway, has trails that are popular with local on-foot exercisers and generally devoid of ambling

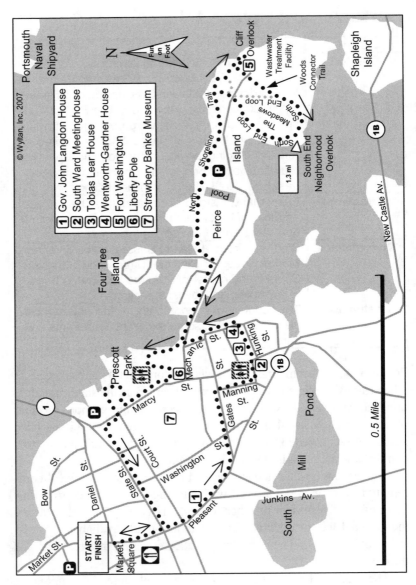

tourists. To get to Peirce Island, assuming a start and finish in the heart of the city at Market Square, we took the simple approach of using one of the Harbor Trail routes. That way, you get the opportunity to soak up a little history while getting to and from the island.

Start in Market Square, and try to pick up a Harbor Trail guide from an information desk before starting out. Follow the green route (South End section) of the Harbor Trail, along Pleasant Street, left into Gates Street, and right into Manning Street to the South Ward Meetinghouse (now the Children's Museum of Portsmouth) at 280 Marcy Street. Cross Marcy Street into Hunking Street, and go left into Mechanic Street to where the causeway to Peirce Island heads off to the right.

Cross to Peirce Island and follow the road past the bridge to Four Tree Island. Bear left and pick up the pedestrian path heading east along the northern shore of Peirce Island. Pass the pool and parking lot and continue to the end of the path at the scenic cliff overlook. Near here are the remains of Fort Washington, built to protect Portsmouth in the American Revolution.

Backtrack about 100 yards to the trail junction where you can follow a trail south across the road near the gate into the Water Treatment Facility. This trail, called the Woods Connector Trail, leads you to the South End Loop Trail, a 0.3-mile loop through a pleasant wooded area on the southern part of Peirce Island. At the trail's southern extremity, there is a spot with a lovely view of Portsmouth's South End.

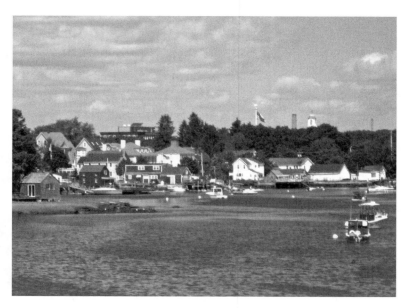

Portsmouth's Quaintness as Viewed from Peirce Island

Continue around the South End Loop Trail back to the road. Follow the road back to mainland Portsmouth at Mechanic Street.

Here pick up the Harbor Trail to the right into Prescott Park. Negotiate Prescott Park following the Harbor Trail guide or make your own route. Eventually you exit onto Marcy Street. Go to the right along Marcy Street to State Street. Turn left into State Street and follow it back to Pleasant Street. Turn right and return to your start point at Market Square.

If you feel the need for a food and beverage break, we can personally recommend the nearby Coat of Arms British Pub at 174 Fleet Street, with its house-made pastry pies. We also liked the Portsmouth Brewery at 56 Market Street.

Portsmouth: New Castle Loop

Distance	6.9 miles
Comfort	This route follows street sidewalks or street edges the entire way. There is significant traffic close by in parts, and care is required of pedestrians. The route is mostly level. Expect to encounter ample other pedestrians on the first half of the route, with fewer on the second half. Not suitable for inline skating.
Attractions	See the lovely island of New Castle, with its relaxed, somewhat exclusive community. There are many scenic views along the way. With short diversions you can see the Fort Constitution and Fort Stark historic sites.
Convenience	Start and finish at Market Square, at the corner of Market Street (or Pleasant Street) and Congress Street in the center of Portsmouth. This is handy to city hotels and tourist attractions.
Destination	The center of Portsmouth, with innumerable historic sites plus some excellent restaurants and bars.

Our second Portsmouth route is more of a challenge than the first, committing you to an outing of almost seven miles. However, it takes you on a very interesting journey from Portsmouth through the nearby island community of New Castle.

From Market Square take Pleasant Street, which is also Route 1B. Route 1B is the highway sign to follow for the first five miles of this route. Pleasant Street merges into Marcy Street, which crosses the sea entrance to South Mill Pond. Then swing left into New Castle Avenue. This road hops across two small islands before launching you into Portsmouth Avenue on New Castle's Great Island.

New Castle is an independent municipality. It is the smallest town in New Hampshire, with an area of 0.8 square miles, or 512 acres. The road through New Castle, for most of its length, does not have sidewalks so pedestrians need to use the road's verge. However, many runners and walkers do just that, so most car drivers are well used to it. In general, use the left side of the road so that you are facing oncoming

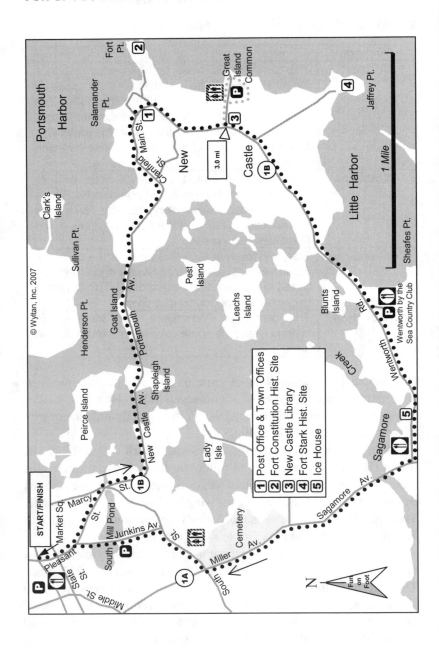

© Wyttan, Inc. 2007

Portsmouth Harbor

Fort Pt. [2]

Salamander Pt.

Great Island Common [4]

Jaffrey Pt.

[1] Main St.

Cranfield St.

New Castle

[3]

3.0 mi

1B

Little Harbor

Sheafes Pt.

1 Mile

Clark's Island

Sullivan Pt.

Goat Island

Portsmouth Av.

Pest Island

Leachs Island

Blunts Island

Wentworth Rd.

Wentworth by the Sea Country Club

P

Henderson Pt.

Shapleigh Island

New Castle Av.

Lady Isle

Creek

Peirce Island

START/FINISH

Marcy St.

1B

St.

Market Sq

South Mill Pond

Junkins Av.

P

St.

Miller Av.

Cemetery

Sagamore Av.

Sagamore Av.

[5]

|1| Post Office & Town Offices
|2| Fort Constitution Hist. Site
|3| New Castle Library
|4| Fort Stark Hist. Site
|5| Ice House

Ice House

Pleasant St.

State St.

Middle St.

1A

South St.

N

Fun on Foot

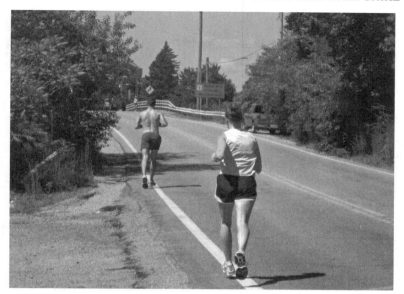

The Road to Newcastle is Popular with Local Runners

traffic. In a few places, where the left verge becomes too narrow, we felt it prudent to cross the road and use the other side.

Continue along Route 1B, which changes name to Cranfield Street and then Main Street. Pass the Post Office and Town Offices. There are several historically preserved houses from the eighteenth century along this stretch as well. At the street to the left with a sign indicating the U.S. Coast Guard Station, you might wish to divert to see historic Fort Constitution. After this, Route 1B changes name again to Wentworth Road.

A short distance further on you come to the Town Library and a street to the left leading to the Great Island Common. It is worthwhile diverting here, especially if you feel the need for a restroom stop. In any case, the Common is worth visiting. It is a pleasant area, with a good beach, sports fields, and playgrounds, very popular with the locals. There are views of two lighthouses.

After the Common, continue south on Route 1B. While the road verge is not the best in this stretch, after a short distance a paved sidewalk starts on the left side of the road. The general character of the environment also changes to up-market residential. You are approaching the Wentworth by the Sea Country Club, a classy hotel and golf resort. If you need a food, beverage, or restroom break, this is the place for that. Nola and I spoke to the concierge and were pleased to learn that he recommends exactly the loop we are describing here to guests who are seeking a good run, jog, or bike ride.

Continue along Route 1B. The next place of interest, especially on a hot day, is the Ice House. It is best known for its ice cream menu but it also serves hot snack food. After that, you pass on your right BG's Boat House, a popular full service restaurant and lounge. You then come to the intersection of Route 1B with Sagamore Avenue or Route 1A. Follow the edge of Route 1A to the right. While this busy road at first appears somewhat unfriendly to the pedestrian, after a few hundred yards a good paved sidewalk starts on the left-hand side and continues to the end of our route.

Follow Route 1A past the cemetery to the traffic light at South Street. Turn right following South Street and then left into Junkins Avenue. Cross the South Mill Pond causeway and continue to where Junkins merges with Pleasant Street. Pleasant Street leads you back to Market Square. For our suggestions re food and beverage places near there, see our first Portsmouth route description.

Lebanon: Northern Rail Trail and Mill Road

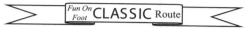

Distance	7.7 miles
Comfort	This route involves 5.3 miles on a paved, well maintained rail trail, 1.6 miles on a gravel untrafficked road, and 0.8 miles on street sidewalks or edges. The 0.4 miles on the edge of Riverside Drive requires some care, since there may be some traffic. The going is level throughout and the entire route is excellent for running. Expect to encounter plenty of other pedestrians on this route. The rail trail is excellent for inline skating, but not River Road, so inline skaters would need to keep to the rail trail.
Attractions	A particularly beautiful trail following the course of the Mascoma River. Both the rail trail and River Road are very pleasant, and using both adds variety on the outbound and return legs. Sights include a covered bridge, which is still in active use.
Convenience	Start and finish at City Hall, opposite Coburn Park, in the center of Lebanon.
Destination	The peaceful center of Lebanon, with a selection of shops, restaurants and bars.

Lebanon, established in 1761, calls itself the Crossroads of New England. That is because Lebanon is located near the intersection of the Interstate 89 and 91 highway systems, at the main gateway point between New Hampshire and Vermont. Lebanon is also a very attractive little city, and has some excellent on-foot trails very close to the city center. The route we are featuring here is so good it scored our Classic Route ribbon.

This route uses a combination of two designated trails, the Northern Rail Trail and Mill Road Trail, both of which follow the course of the Mascoma River. The Northern Rail Trail extends 23 miles, through Enfield, Canaan, Orange, and Grafton. We chose, however, to go just four miles up the river, to a point just below the junction of highways 4

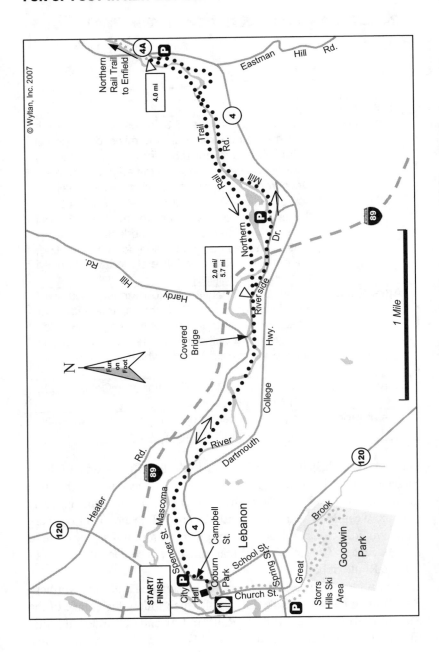

and 4A—a convenient turnaround point that allows you to make best use of both trails.

Colburn Park is the center of Lebanon, with City Hall across the street. Start here. Go up Campbell Street a block and turn left into Spencer Street. This brings you to the trailhead for the Northern Rail Trail.

This is an excellent rail trail, very popular with the locals. We passed many runners, walkers, dog-walkers, baby-walkers, and, quite surprisingly, no bicycles (although they are permitted). The trail is maintained by the all-volunteer Friends of the Northern Rail Trail.

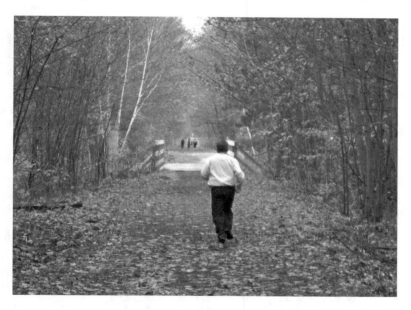

The Northern Rail Trail in Fall

The trail crosses the river several times before reaching Riverside Drive. Just before the Riverside Drive intersection you pass a covered bridge—quite impressive, given the small number of covered bridges in active use today.

At Riverside Drive, leave the rail trail and follow the street to the right, using the left verge of the road. We experienced very little traffic and felt the verge was quite wide enough for the short distance involved, but you should take care. Go under Interstate 89 to where Mill

Road branches off to the left with its Dead End sign. Follow the road a short distance to where the trafficable road abruptly ends and there is a gate declaring the start of the Mill Road Trail. Mill Road was once a vehicle road, but is now reserved for unmotorized activities. It is a spectacularly beautiful trail, following the southern bank of the river, with little babbling streams and waterfalls along the way. It is actually more beautiful than the rail trail, so being able to combine these two trails is a particularly attractive option.

Follow Mill Road to where it meets and runs parallel to the rail trail for about a hundred yards. At this point, keep to Mill Road.

VARIATION
If you want to cut the route short by about a mile, take this opportunity to turn around and follow the rail trail back to Lebanon center.

Mill Road continues up the river and we found this last part the most scenic. Eventually you come to a trailhead where the road opens up for traffic again. A little further on you come to a path down to the rail trail. This is immediately before the junction of Mill Road with Route 4, which is also the junction of Routes 4 and 4A.

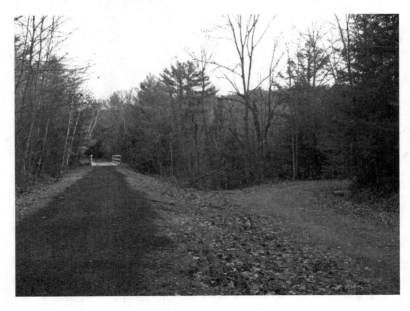

The Northern Rail Trail and Mill Road Meet

Take the rail trail to the left. Shortly after going under the Interstate-89 overpass, you arrive back at Riverside Road. Retrace your steps back to Lebanon center.

If you feel like a food and beverage break after your on-foot outing, we can recommend the Salt Hill Pub, a down-home Irish pub with good food. It is across from the western end of Coburn Park. We also like the nearby Three Tomatoes Italian restaurant.

Other Routes

We discussed routes in easy on-foot reach of central **Concord** in our featured routes above. However, there are some good on-foot trails a little further out from the city center. Of particular note are the **Oak Hill Trails**, roughly five miles north of the city center. There are about seven miles of trails here, used for multiple purposes including training for the local high school cross country running team. There are also several miles of trails in **Mast Yard State Forest** and nearby on the Contoocook River—this area is about seven miles west of central Concord, near the city's boundary with **Hopkinton**.[5]

Hanover, home of Dartmouth College, is a charming town, about five miles up the Connecticut River from Interstate 89 and Lebanon. There are several comparatively short, but pleasant trails close to the town center. They include a 2.7-mile walk featuring Old Houses of Hanover, a 1.7-mile loop of Pine Park, a protected natural area a mile north of the town center, and a 1.8-mile loop of Storrs Pond, about two miles north of town. These and other trails around Hanover and Lebanon have been nicely documented by the Upper Valley Trails Alliance.[6]

The city of **Keene** has an active running community, and a map of local trails can be purchased from local stores or by mail.[7] Most notably, Keene is the hub of an impressive rail-trail system. The longest trail is the **Cheshire Branch Rail Trail**, stretching north through **Walpole** to **Cold River** and southeast through **Troy** to **Winchendon**. The other major trail is the **Ashuelot Rail Trail**, stretching southwest through **Swanzey** and **Winchester** to **Hinsdale**. Pieces of these trails are still being filled in. Keene also has some good trails around the city center. The **Ashuelot River Trail** stretches roughly a mile through Ashuelot River Park and connects at its northern end to the **Appel Way Trail** to Wheelock Park. From there you can follow local streets south to downtown and take the **Downtown Cheshire Trail** back to the river, thereby completing a roughly three-mile loop.

We earlier featured one outstanding route in **Lebanon**. This city has some other on-foot routes, a particularly interesting one being **Goodwin**

---

5   The Concord trail system is largely attributable to the Groundwork Concord organization (See: http://www.groundworkconcord.org) and the City of Concord (See: http://www.onconcord.com). Refer to these sites for more details.
6   See: http://www.uvtrails.org
7   See: http://www.tlaorg.org/pathways/pathmap.html

Park, which is 0.55 mile from Coburn Park. You can do a nice 4.1-mile Fun-on-Foot route from and back to the city center; this is ideal for a lunchtime escape if you want a change from the rail trail. From Coburn Park, go down Church Street, turn right into Spring Street, and then cross the bridge to the ski area car park on the left. Here you find the start of Goodwin Park's three-mile exercise trail loop. It involves nice unpaved trails through the woods, close to a running stream (the Great Brook), well away from people and traffic. There was once a series of exercise stations here, but those exercise stations and their signage have deteriorated to the point of uselessness. Nevertheless, it is still a good place for on-foot exercise.

About five miles east of **Manchester** is **Massabesic Lake**, which has several trails around and near it. You can obtain a trail map from the Massabesic Audubon Center.[8] This is near the town of **Auburn**.

Massabesic Lake is also the western end of a 25-mile rail trail, called the **Portsmouth Branch Rail Trail**, which loosely follows Route 101 through **Raymond** and **Epping** to **Newfields**, near the Atlantic coast. There is actually a network of interesting rail trails around here. The 18-mile **Rockingham Recreational Trail** stretches south from **Epping**, through **Fremont** and **Sandown** to **Windham Depot** near Interstate 93. Windham Depot is also on the **Derry Rail Trail**, giving on-foot access to the cities of **Derry** and **Salem**. With some planning, there is enormous potential to craft interesting Fun-on-Foot routes around here. To gain a good appreciation of the geography of these and other New Hampshire long-haul trails, I recommend the New Hampshire Topaz Outdoor Travel Map.[9]

Another nice trail in the Manchester-Auburn region is the roughly four-mile loop of **Tower Hill Pond**. From Massabesic Lake, head east on the Portsmouth Branch Rail Trail about two miles to the branch path heading north, under Route 101, to Tower Hill Pond.

Mount Washington, at 6,288 feet, is the highest mountain in New England, and the center of an outstanding summer and winter resort area. We found some excellent summer running, jogging, walking trails near the majestic Mount Washington Resort Hotel at **Bretton Woods**. Start from the Mount Washington Hotel, where you can pick up a free trail map from the hotel's "adventure center." The trails here double as

8   See: http://www.nhaudubon.org/sanctuaries/massabesic.htm
9   See: http://www.topazmaps.com

winter Nordic trails and are accordingly graded green, blue, and black. Anything green or blue is suitable for running, except possibly for the occasional steeper spot. The trails are quite well signposted. For a loop of about five miles, start out along the bridle path (sometimes signposted as the bridal path). Follow the river until you meet the B&M trail, named after the Boston & Maine railroad that ran through here a long time ago. Pass a small shelter on the left. Turn right onto the Coronary Hills trail. The first part of this is a substantial uphill, but the second part is downhill all the way back to the hotel. There are also both longer and shorter trail options in this beautiful trail system.

The **Nashua River Rail Trail** is a paved trail stretching 11.2 miles from **Nashua** to Ayer, Massachusetts, through the Massachusetts centers of Dunstable, Pepperell, and Groton.[10]

We described the Lebanon end of the **Northern Rail Trail** in our featured route. This trail, however, stretches 23 miles from Lebanon, through **Enfield**, **Canaan**, **Orange**, and **Grafton**, almost to **Danbury**. The long-term plan is for a 65-mile trail from Concord to Vermont. For details, refer to the Friends of the Northern Rail Trail.[11]

The **Sugar River Recreational Trail** is a 10-mile rail trail connecting **Newport** and **Claremont**. For more details, see *The Official Rails-to-Trails Conservancy Guidebook.*[12]

As usual, we have not tried to cover serious hiking trails, as distinct from trails we feel will appeal to local or visiting runners, joggers, and walkers. New Hampshire has more than its fair share of serious hiking experiences, including the **Appalachian Trail**, the various hikes up **Mount Washington**, and the hikes up scenic 3,165-foot **Mount Monadnock**. The latter is claimed to be the most climbed mountain in the world. Please enjoy these experiences too.

---

10   See: http://www.mass.gov/dcr/parks/northeast/nash.htm
11   See: http://www.northernrailtrail.org
12   By Cynthia Mascott, 2000, published by The Globe Pequot Press.

9

Ocean State: Rhode Island

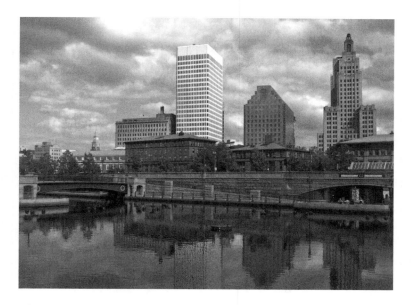

T he 13th state, Rhode Island, is the nation's tiniest state, with an area of only 1,214 square miles. However, its population is just a little under that of New Hampshire and it contains New England's second-largest city, Providence.

Having such a small land area, the size of a square 35 miles by 35 miles, it is somewhat surprising to note that Rhode Island reputedly has over 400 miles of coastline.

With all its coastline and waterways, it is less surprising that Rhode Island is a popular tourist destination and a popular place for outdoor exercise. Furthermore, the state and its community take very seriously the need for pedestrian and bicycle trails. We introduce some of these trails in this chapter.

If you want to use public transit to get to or from exercise routes, there is a statewide bus network operated by The Rhode Island Public Transit Authority (RIPTA). The bus services are inexpensive and generally comfortable, and mostly run seven days a week. RIPTA operates trolley services around downtown Providence.

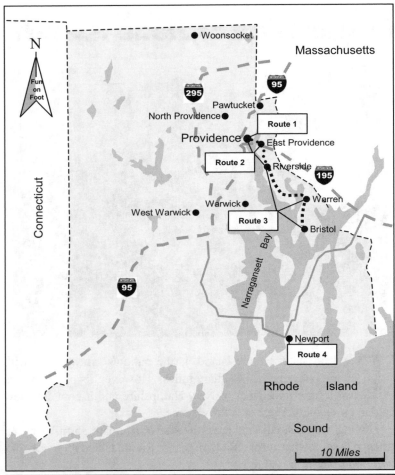

1.	Providence: Blackstone Boulevard (3.2 or 6.4 miles)
2.	Riverside-E Providence-Providence: East Bay Bike Path (4.0 or 5.4 miles)
3.	Riverside-Warren-Bristol: East Bay Bike Path (5.8 or 10.0 miles)
4.	Newport: Cliff Walk and Bellevue (6.9 miles)

Rhode Island Featured Routes

Providence: Blackstone Boulevard

Distance	3.2 or 6.4 miles
Comfort	Half of this route is on street sidewalks and half on a pleasant pedestrian trail along the wide, beautifully landscaped nature strip of a lightly trafficked suburban road. Expect plenty of other people sharing the trail, including runners, joggers, and walkers. Suitable for inline skating in parts but not overall.
Attractions	The natural beauty of a well-landscaped trail. Pass through the district surrounding the Brown University campus.
Convenience	Start and finish in downtown Providence, close to the Convention Center and most downtown hotels. If you want to limit your on-foot outing to 3.2 miles, use a RIPTA bus for the return segment.
Destination	Downtown Providence, close to good pub/restaurants, the Riverwalk, Providence Place Mall, and historic attractions.

Blackstone Boulevard is Providence's most popular running place. It has 1.7 miles of comfortable paved trail along the center of a wide, nicely landscaped nature strip in a suburban setting. It is handy to the Brown University campus. It is a little further from downtown, but you can still easily get there on-foot.

To accommodate downtown workers or visitors, we assume a start at Burnside Park, adjacent to the Kennedy Plaza Transportation Center, and convenient to the convention center and most downtown hotels.

From the north corner of the park, at Exchange Terrace and Exchange Street, go down Exchange Terrace and cross busy Memorial Boulevard, coming to the Steeple Street bridge across the Providence River. Cross the river, and continue up Steeple Street, which becomes Saint Thomas Street. The going is a little steep here, but only for a short distance. Saint Thomas Street becomes Angell Street. Follow Angell Street through the Brown University campus and past Brown's Aldrich-Dexter field. There are various shops on this street and possibly a lot of ambling pedestrians; if this bothers you, go a block south and follow Waterman Street, which is less busy.

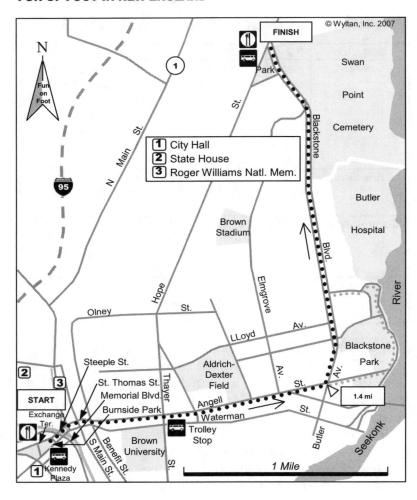

When you come to the intersection with Butler Avenue, turn left. Butler Avenue leads into Blackstone Boulevard.

VARIATION

If you continue straight on Angell Street, it takes you into Blackstone Park, a leafy park with the bank of the Seekonk River its eastern boundary. Go through the park and up the eastern edge along the river. Continue to where you are forced to turn back inland. The streets will take you back to Blackstone Boulevard. This variation adds a little variety to your outing, plus about a half-mile in distance.

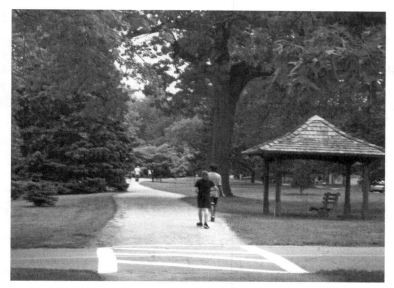

The Blackstone Boulevard Trail

Blackstone Boulevard's conditions for running, jogging, or walking are outstanding, and the local residents reward it with the popularity it deserves. There is a wide reserve down the middle of the street, with an excellent path, trees and other landscaping. Expect plenty of pedestrians here, but the reserve is sufficiently wide that crowds are unlikely to be a concern. You need to cross a few cross-streets but the custom here is that vehicles give way to pedestrians using the trail.

Continue to the end of the trail at Hope Street. You have various options as to what to do next. If 3.2 miles is enough for you, there are a few restaurants and food joints around here (including some with Sunday brunch) and you can catch a bus on the west side of Hope Street back to downtown.

If 6.4 miles is more to your liking, use your feet to get back downtown. While there are different route options, such as Hope Street, the most pleasant approach is probably to retrace your outbound route on Blackstone Boulevard.

When you get back to Burnside Park or Kennedy Plaza, if you want a food and beverage break there are some excellent places around here. Just north of Burnside Park, in what used to be the old Union Station complex, there are some good pub/restaurants. Nola and I always end up in Ri Ra Irish Pub here.

If you are a visitor to Providence, you should also be aware of the Riverwalk, which is a series of pedestrian pathways along the canal and the river. Unfortunately, the Riverwalk is not of much value as a place to exercise, since it is not long enough and is often crowded. However, it can be an outstanding evening entertainment area. On Saturday nights, a chain of fires is lit in baskets in the middle of the canal and river, and music from around the world is played, lending a unique atmosphere and attracting many people. Nola and I will never forget a Halloween evening we spent here, wandering among the costumed and the un-costumed in the eerie light and sampling the wares of the nearby food and beverage establishments.

The Riverwalk terminates in Waterplace Park, across the water from the Union Station complex.

If you are into sightseeing, in short walking distance of here you will find the State House and the National Memorial to Roger Williams, founder of Rhode Island's first European settlement in 1636. If you are into shopping, the Providence Place Mall is nearby.

Riverside-E Providence-Providence: East Bay Bike Path

Distance	4.0 or 5.4 miles
Comfort	Four miles on a well-maintained paved multi-use trail. If the Washington Bridge pedestrian walkway is open, continue along sidewalks and pedestrian areas to downtown Providence. If the walkway is not open, either retrace steps or catch a bus downtown from near the bridge in East Providence. On a nice day expect plenty of other pedestrians and cyclists on the same route. Generally OK for inline skating.
Attractions	Scenic views of the Providence River estuary, parks, and the Providence skyline.
Convenience	Catch a bus from downtown Providence to the start in Riverside. Finish in downtown Providence, close to the Convention Center and most downtown hotels. If the Washington Bridge pedestrian walkway is not open, you will need to catch a bus from East Providence to downtown. Buses run daily but are not very frequent so you should consult timetables in advance.
Destination	Downtown Providence, close to good pub/restaurants, the Riverwalk, Providence Place Mall, and historic attractions.

The East Bay Bike Path, a 14.2-mile rail trail from central Providence to the attractive seaport town of Bristol, is an outstanding resource. While designed with cyclists forefront in mind, it offers outstanding conditions for on-footers too, and you will find many runners, joggers, and walkers on this trail.

To address the most attractive options for pedestrians, we have split the trail into two parts. In this first route, we cover the northern 4.2 miles of the trail from Riverside to the Washington Bridge, which connects Providence and East Providence. Adding on 1.2 miles from the bridge to downtown makes the total distance 5.4 miles.

Provided the Washington Bridge pedestrian walkway is open, we have an excellent route, ending downtown, which satisfies all of our Fun-on-Foot route criteria well. In fact, in a few years time, I am

FUN OF FOOT IN NEW ENGLAND

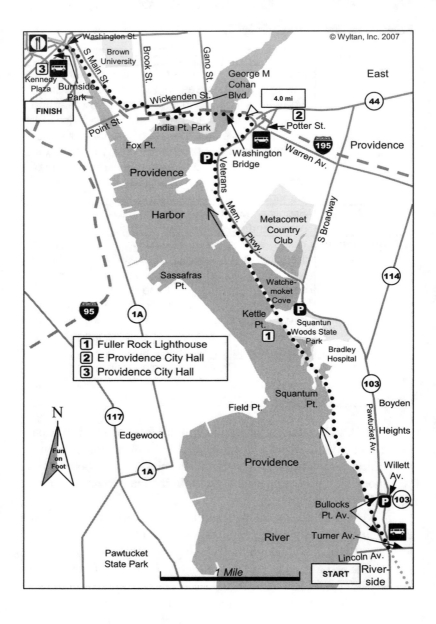

© Wyltan, Inc. 2007

Washington St.
Brown University
S Main St.
Brook St.
Gano St.
George M Cohan Blvd.
East
Kennedy Plaza
Burnside Park
Wickenden St.
4.0 mi
44
FINISH
Point St.
India Pt. Park
Potter St.
Providence
Fox Pt.
Washington Bridge
Warren Av.
195
Providence
Veterans
Harbor
Mem. Pkwy.
Metacomet Country Club
S Broadway
Sassafras Pt.
Watche-moket Cove
114
Kettle Pt.
Squantun Woods State Park
95
1A
Bradley Hospital
1 Fuller Rock Lighthouse
2 E Providence City Hall
3 Providence City Hall
103
N
117
Field Pt.
Squantum Pt.
Boyden
Edgewood
Heights
Fun on Foot
1A
Providence
Willett Av.
Pawtucket Av.
Bullocks Pt. Av.
103
Pawtucket State Park
River
Turner Av.
1 Mile
Lincoln Av.
START
River-side

expecting to be able to designate this a Classic Route. The reason for the delay is that the Rhode Island Department of Transport (RIDOT) is in the process of major modifications to the bridge. One of the planned results is a feature called the Washington Bridge Linear Park, a wide bridge detached from the highway structure and dedicated to pedestrians and bicycles. It will connect to the East Bay Bike Path at the East Providence end and India Point Park at the Providence end. The plans look very impressive.

At the time of writing, that facility is not built, but there is a functional (although not particularly attractive) pedestrian and bike sidewalk on the highway bridge that satisfies our main purpose.

Unfortunately, there is a catch. My quizzing of the helpful RIDOT engineers suggests there will likely be a period of two-to-five years in which there will be no pedestrian or bicycle access over the Washington Bridge at all, because of the construction process. During that period, our enthusiasm for this route must drop, but not completely go away. The top four miles of the East Bay Bike Path will still be a beautiful place to run or walk, and there will be an option to catch a bus over the bridge from near its East Providence end.

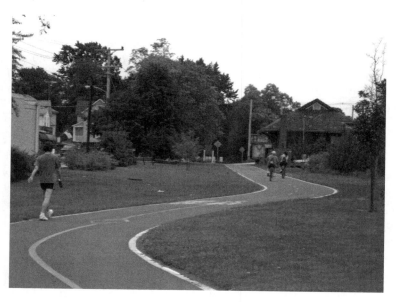

East Bay Bike Path at Riverside

The main message here is that, before setting out to run or walk across the Washington Bridge, please check current status at the RIDOT website.[1]   Also, if you decide to use the bus, note that it may not be particularly frequent, so check out the timetable in advance.[2]

To get to Riverside, you can drive and park or you can catch the Riverside bus from Kennedy Plaza in downtown Providence. The bus route mainly follows Route 103 but when that route takes a sharp left into Willett Avenue, the bus continues straight ahead into Bullocks Point Avenue and the little center of Riverside. The road crosses the bike path and follows it for a few blocks, so you should alight anywhere here and follow that bike path north.

This part of the trail has some very attractive parts, since it largely hugs the shoreline. You do not need our directions now—the path is well defined and signposted, including mile and half-mile markers. Relax and enjoy the pleasant on-foot environment.

After crossing the causeway at Watchemoket Cove, the trail leaves the rail bed and generally follows Veterans Memorial Parkway to the Washington Bridge.

VARIATION

If the bridge walkway is closed and you want to take a bus downtown from here, you need to get onto Warren Avenue, the main street before and parallel to the Interstate. Go under Veterans Memorial Parkway, find Warren Avenue, and find the intersection with Potter Street. Here there is a stop for the bus with a destination of downtown Providence.

If you can walk across Washington Bridge, do so and exit the bridge walkway onto the elevated walkway above India Point Park. This park is also popular with pedestrians. Cross the Interstate using the new pedestrian overpass, scheduled for opening in 2008. (If that overpass is not yet open, go down to street level and use Gano Street.) Find Wickenden Street. There are some basic food and beverage places here if you need that by now.

Follow Wickenden Street to the west and go right into Main Street. Go down to the river walkway and follow the river to the Washington Street Bridge. Cross the river and go straight ahead to Burnside Park,

1   See: http://www.dot.state.ri.us/bikeri
2   See: http://www.ripta.com

Kennedy Plaza, and the nearby establishments and attractions we discussed in the previous route description.

If you want to terminate your route in Riverside instead of downtown Providence, there are some basic food and beverage places plus other services here.

Riverside-Warren-Bristol: East Bay Bike Path

Distance	5.8 or 10.0 miles
Comfort	The entire route is on a well-maintained paved multi-use trail. The going is level and there are few traffic intersections. Parts of the trail are shady. There are services at various points along the way. On a nice day expect plenty of other pedestrians and cyclists on the same route. Good for inline skating.
Attractions	A pleasant escape from traffic and crowds, passing through a variety of environments. There are some stretches with scenic bayside views, some shady tree-lined stretches, and some stretches skirting pleasant towns.
Convenience	Catch a bus from downtown Providence to the start in Riverside. Finish in the center of either Warren or Bristol. Both of these places are on the Providence-Newport bus route, so you can conveniently catch a bus to either major center. Buses run daily but are not necessarily frequent so you should consult timetables in advance.
Destination	Bristol is a winning destination, with a choice of restaurant/bars overlooking the scenic Bristol Harbor and a quaint town center with a variety of small shops. Warren is an alternative destination, with a couple of reasonable food and beverage establishments and basic services. Catch a bus to Providence or Newport from either.

We covered the northern 4.2 miles of the East Bay Bike path in our previous route. Here we cover the remaining ten miles, from Riverside to Bristol, or you can cut that short by finishing the route in Warren. To get to Riverside by bus, follow the same directions as for the previous route.

The segment of the rail trail from Riverside to Warren is more inland than both the northern segment and the Warren to Bristol segment, and tends to be green, shady, and pleasant throughout. You pass through Haines Memorial State Park, which offers the luxury of seasonal

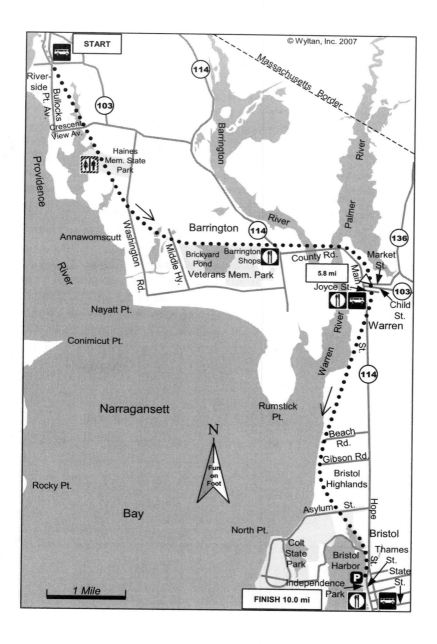

START

© Wyltan, Inc. 2007

114

Massachusetts Border

Riverside Pt. Av.
Bullocks Pt. Av.
103

Crescent View Av.

Barrington River

River

Palmer River

Haines Mem. State Park

Providence River

Annawomscutt

Washington Rd.
Middle Hy.

Barrington
114

River

136

Brickyard Pond
Barrington Shops
County Rd.
Market St.

Veterans Mem. Park

5.8 mi

Main St.

Joyce St.

103

Child St.

Warren

Nayatt Pt.

Warren River

St.

Conimicut Pt.

114

Narragansett

Rumstick Pt.

N

Beach Rd.

Gibson Rd.

Bristol Highlands

Fun on Foot

Rocky Pt.

Asylum St.

Hope St.

Bay

North Pt.

Bristol

Colt State Park

Thames St.

Bristol Harbor

State St.

1 Mile

Independence Park

FINISH 10.0 mi

249

restrooms. (There are no other restrooms on the route, although there are commercial businesses at a few points that might allow you to use their facilities in an emergency.)

At 4.5 miles from Riverside, you pass the Barrington Shopping Center. You can stop here for emergency supplies if needed. Shortly after that, you cross two dedicated pedestrian/bicycle bridges, over the Barrington River and Palmer River, respectively.

You then pass by the center of Warren, about a block away from its Main Street. If you have had enough on-foot activity and want to catch a bus to Providence or Newport, here is a good place to do that. Leave the bike path where it intersects Market Street or Child Street, and follow either of those streets west one block to Main Street. There is a choice of cafes and restaurants for a food or beverage break. The bus stop for the Providence-Newport RIPTA bus is at the intersection of Main Street and Joyce Street.

Bristol is an even better place to end an on-foot route. The trail continues 4.2 miles from Warren to Bristol via a route that hugs the scenic shore of Narragansett Bay for part of the way. The trail terminates in Independence Park on the edge of Bristol Harbor. From the park, proceed a block further south along Thames Street and you come to a selection of restaurants, cafes, and bars on the shore of the attractive harbor. This is an ideal place for a well-earned break after a good exercise outing. When ready, proceed inland one block to Hope Street, Bristol's main street, where the shops are clustered. The bus stop for the Providence-Newport RIPTA bus is at the intersection of Hope Street and State Street.

VARIATION

If you happen to be staying near Warren or Bristol, simply run, jog, or walk the 4.2 miles from one place to the other. Then either return on foot or catch the Providence-Newport bus back to where you started.

If using the bus, be sure to check out a timetable in advance, especially on Sundays when bus frequency is questionable.

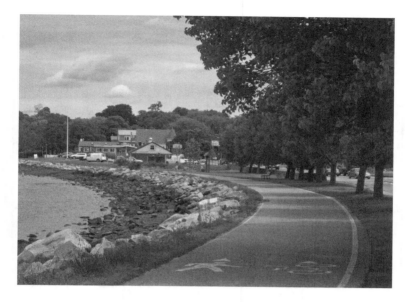

The East Bay Bike Path Near its Bristol End

Newport: Cliff Walk and Bellevue

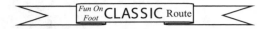

Distance	6.9 miles
Comfort	The Cliff Walk comprises 3.5 miles of this route. The northern part of the Cliff Walk is an excellent paved trail, well suited to running. The southern part includes rocky paths with the occasional steep grade. The remaining 3.4 miles are along good street sidewalks. Expect to encounter many other pedestrians, mostly strolling sightseers but also some athletes, on all parts of this route. Not suitable for inline skating.
Attractions	Some of the most spectacular scenery you will find anywhere, including rocky cliffs, breaking waves, and numerous awe-inspiring mansions. On the return leg via Bellevue Avenue, you pass more mansions and other historic attractions.
Convenience	Start and end in the center of Newport. You can get to Newport from Providence by RIPTA ferry (seasonal), RIPTA bus, or car.
Destination	The center of Newport, with innumerable attractions plus several excellent restaurants and bars.

Newport is about 25 miles south of Providence and can be reached by ferry (seasonal), bus, or car. Newport is well known for various reasons. Founded in 1639, it was a major seaport for much of its existence. Its colorful history, which includes its role as a major summer retreat for wealthy New Yorkers in the nineteenth century, has left Newport with some of the most impressive architecture and preserved buildings in the country. It is now an extremely popular tourist destination. It was once famous as the long-term host port for America's Cup races. For the on-footer, it is well known for the Cliff Walk, one of the most popular on-foot trails in the country. No book on New England on-foot outings could be complete without covering the Cliff Walk.

We have put together a loop that includes the entire Cliff Walk, with a return via Bellevue Avenue, the street on which many of the famous Newport mansions are located. Much of the route is suitable for running.

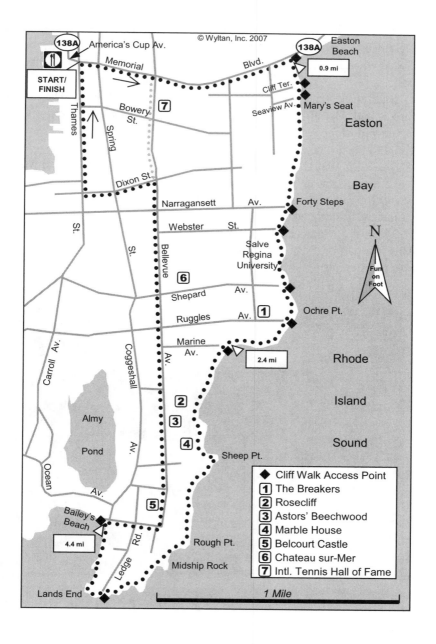

138A
America's Cup Av.
© Wyltan, Inc. 2007
138A
Easton Beach
0.9 mi

START/ FINISH

Memorial
Blvd.
Cliff Ter.
Seaview Av.
Mary's Seat

Thames
Bowery St.
7
Spring

Easton

Dixon St.
Narragansett Av.
Forty Steps

Bay

Webster St.

St.
St.
Bellevue
Salve Regina University

N

6
Shepard Av.
Ruggles Av.
1
Ochre Pt.

Fun on Foot

Carroll Av.
Coggeshall
Av.
Marine Av.
2.4 mi

Rhode

2
3

Island

Almy Pond
Av.
4
Sheep Pt.

Sound

Ocean Av.
5
Bailey's Beach
4.4 mi

Cliff Walk Access Point
1 The Breakers
2 Rosecliff
3 Astors' Beechwood
4 Marble House
5 Belcourt Castle
6 Chateau sur-Mer
7 Intl. Tennis Hall of Fame

Ledge Rd.
Rough Pt.
Midship Rock

Lands End

1 Mile

The southernmost parts of the Cliff Walk involve clambering over rocks in parts, but the scenery there is so spectacular it is worth negotiating regardless. One caution: Parts of the Cliff Walk may sometimes be closed when Lyme disease ticks or poison ivy plants are present on the trail.

Start at the center of town, where America's Cup Avenue, Thames Street, and Memorial Boulevard meet. Head east along Memorial Boulevard to the water, with the view of Easton's Beach ahead. Here you find the trailhead for the Cliff Walk.

The Cliff Walk has many points of interest along the way, and we make no attempt to mention them all. For more details, refer to the www.cliffwalk.com website[3] or the Cliff Walk and Bellevue Avenue Guide and Touring Map.[4]

From the Memorial Boulevard trailhead, follow the trail south. This first part of the trail is paved and in excellent condition. It is suitable for running. Bikes are not permitted.

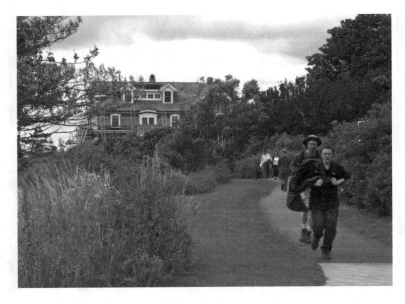

Northern Part of the Cliff Walk

---

3   See: http://www.cliffwalk.com
4   See: http://www.cliffwalk.com/map.htm

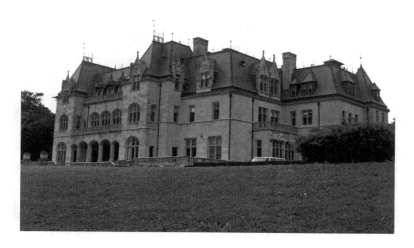

Ochre Court, Now Part of Salve Regina University

At Narragansett Avenue, you find the Forty Steps, a stone staircase leading down the cliffs to a platform overlooking the sea. The next stretch, to Ruggles Avenue, is mostly along the edge of Salve Regina University, which itself occupies four historic mansions. South of the university is The Breakers, one of the most famous mansions, built by Cornelius Vanderbilt.

Up to Ruggles Avenue the trail is paved, level, and excellent for running. After Ruggles, the going gets more difficult. If you are in serious running training, exit the Cliff Walk here.

Continue to Marine Avenue, where there is a small surfing beach. Marine Avenue is the last exit point for 1.5 miles. The next stretch is very picturesque, but the going is highly varied. You pass various mansions. They include Rosecliff, the 1902-vintage regal white mansion where The Great Gatsby was filmed in 1973. Then there is the Astors' Beechwood mansion, followed by the Marble House and its accompanying Chinese Tea House, directly above the trail.

Eventually you come to Ledge Road and a trail access point. However, at this stage, you may as well complete the trail around to its end at Bellevue Avenue, near Bailey's Beach.

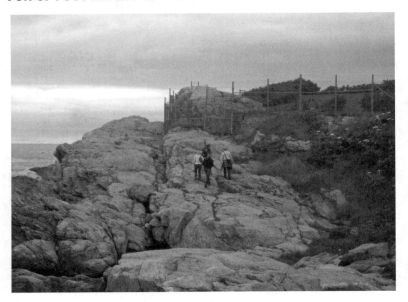

Going Gets Tougher on the Southern Cliff Walk

VARIATION

If you want to lengthen your run by about five miles, head west from Bailey's Beach on Ocean Avenue to Brenton Point State Park. There are various ways to return to downtown Newport from that point.

Follow Bellevue Avenue eastward to where it does a right-angle turn to the left, heading north all the way back to Memorial Boulevard. Many of the mansions front onto Bellevue Avenue, including several that are open to the public. Expect plenty of pedestrians around here on a nice day.

To add a little variety to this route, we chose to divert you to the left at Dixon Street, taking you to Thames Street, Newport's main shopping street. Follow Thames Street north past the many quaint shops to where you started at Memorial Boulevard.

VARIATION

If you have no interest in the shops, keep on Bellevue Avenue back to Memorial Boulevard. There are more historic buildings on this part of Bellevue.

If you need a food or beverage break after your on-foot outing, there are many restaurants and bars in Newport. Nola and I like Buskers Irish Pub and Restaurant and the Brick Alley Pub and Restaurant. We found a mix of locals and visitors in these establishments, and had a lot of fun.

Other Routes

Providence is an excellent city to explore on-foot. The **Providence Banner Trail** is a self-guided walking tour of the city's historic sites. You can pick up a guide map at tourist information desks. Such tourist routes are not, however, particularly useful for exercise purposes.

Roger Williams Park is a 430-acre park embracing a series of attractive lakes, south of downtown Providence. It contains the Museum of Natural History and the zoo. There are various walking and running trails here.

The **Washington Secondary Bike Path** is part of the planned East-Coast Greenway system. Southwest of Providence, it stretches from **Cranston**, through **West Warwick**, to **Coventry**, where it will soon connect to the Coventry Greenway. There are plans for future extensions but, unfortunately, the critical link to downtown Providence is not on the immediate horizon.

The **Blackstone River Bikeway**, north of Providence, currently stretches from **Lincoln** to **Cumberland**. There are plans to extend the southern end down to Pawtucket, eventually linking up with Blackstone Boulevard in Providence. There are longer-term plans to extend the northern end through Woonsocket to link up with the Blackstone River Bikeway in Massachusetts, eventually going to Worcester, Massachusetts.

In **Kingston**, in the south of Rhode Island, the paved 4.3-mile South County Bike Path makes good use of an old rail bed from Kingston Station to Peace Dale.[5]

Work is in progress building a 4.4-mile multi-purpose **Woonasquatucket River Greenway** from Providence's Waterplace Park northwest to the Providence-Johnston border.

* * * *

While Rhode Island is the tiniest state, it is in no way short of interesting places to see or of great places for on-foot exercise. Enjoy the Ocean State!

---

[5]   See *The Official Rails-to-Trails Conservancy Guidebook* by Cynthia Mascott, 2000, published by The Globe Pequot Press.

10

Green Mountain State: Vermont

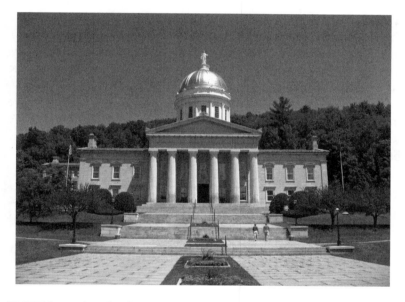

The region that is now Vermont was first visited by a European in 1609, when Samuel de Champlain trekked down from Quebec, giving Lake Champlain its name. Not much happened then until the 18th century, when English settlers started to move in. Up until the American Revolution, the area's status was contentious, subject to competing claims from the colonies of New York and New Hampshire. At the time of the American Revolution, the local people, under the leadership of such individuals as Ethan Allen, fought the British and also succeeded in establishing Vermont as an independent state. In

1791, Vermont was finally admitted as the 14th state of the Union, long after the original 13 states adopted the constitution.

Vermont, a heavily wooded and mountainous area sandwiched between the Connecticut River and Lake Champlain, is a beautiful place. Far removed from the hectic lifestyles of places like Boston and New York, it is an excellent place to live or to visit. The people are all very laid back, and I always notice a kinship to the culture of Canada, not far away to the north. There is also plenty of opportunity to get outdoors and have Fun on Foot, without having to be overly concerned about such factors as traffic, crowds, and crime.

With the second-smallest population of all states (Wyoming has a slightly smaller population), one thing that Vermont does not have much of is urban civilization. The only place remotely resembling a metropolis is the city of Burlington and its surrounding community. The only other city that is a significant destination for visitors is the state's capital, Montpelier.

Therefore, given this book's underlying criteria, we did not have many places we could cover—just Burlington and Montpelier. We feature four routes in these cities, and leave the exploration of the beautiful rural regions of the state to you.

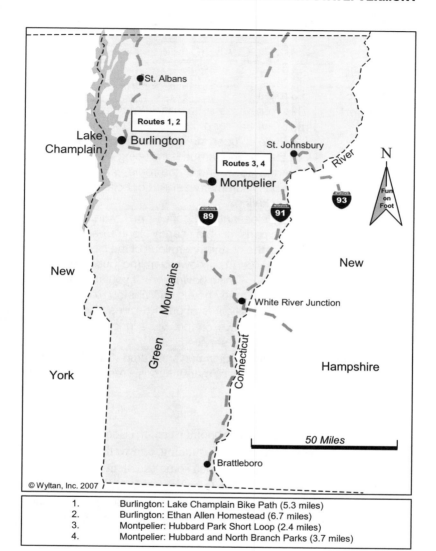

1.	Burlington: Lake Champlain Bike Path (5.3 miles)
2.	Burlington: Ethan Allen Homestead (6.7 miles)
3.	Montpelier: Hubbard Park Short Loop (2.4 miles)
4.	Montpelier: Hubbard and North Branch Parks (3.7 miles)

Vermont Featured Routes

Burlington: Lake Champlain Bike Path

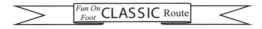

Distance	5.3 miles
Comfort	This route uses a beautifully maintained, paved, multi-use trail for 4.5 miles, with the remainder of the route on good street sidewalks. Expect plenty of other people around, including many joggers. The downtown end of the route can be crowded on a busy summer weekend or holiday. Good for inline skating.
Attractions	A very pleasant and popular trail, with some very scenic parts, such as sandy North Beach.
Convenience	Start at the northern terminus of the North Avenue bus service from downtown (no bus service on Sundays). Finish downtown. If you are staying at one of the many hotels on Williston Road beyond the University, it is about 1.5 miles each way to/from downtown on-foot via a good sidewalk, or there is a bus service.
Destination	Downtown Burlington's Church Street Marketplace, with its many shops, restaurants, and pubs.

Burlington, Vermont's largest metropolitan center, is located on the edge of scenic Lake Champlain. Cycling, running, and walking are popular activities, and the region has developed some excellent off-street trails.

The Lake Champlain Bike Path (also known as the Burlington Bike Path) is seven miles of paved, shared-use rail-trail along the lakeshore through Burlington, starting about 2.5 miles south of Main Street and continuing to about 4.5 miles north of Main Street. These seven miles are actually part of a longer trail continuing further north following the rail bed of the Island Line railroad, a spectacular route spanning several island towns. Ongoing work continues to fill in gaps in that trail.

For a featured route for on-footers based in downtown Burlington, we decided to cover the part of the bike trail north of downtown, and to show how to do it starting with an outbound bus trip from downtown to

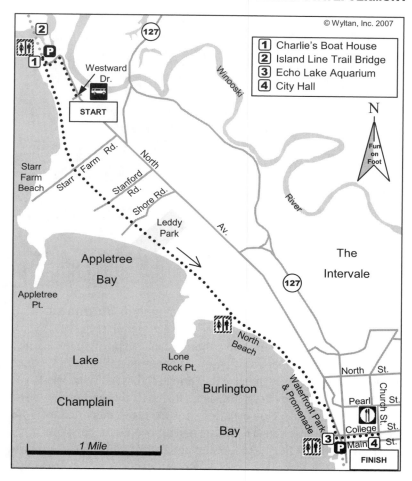

© Wyltan, Inc. 2007

1 Charlie's Boat House
2 Island Line Trail Bridge
3 Echo Lake Aquarium
4 City Hall

the northern start point. Putting all this together, with a finish in lively Church Street Marketplace, makes it a Classic Route to our minds.

Starting from downtown, take the North Avenue bus from Cherry Street to its northern end at Westward Drive. The bus runs with a 30-minute frequency all days except Sunday. On Sundays, the Burlington bus network virtually shuts down. We look forward to them overcoming this eccentricity some day, hopefully soon.

Walk up North Avenue a short distance and follow it around to the left. You quickly intersect the bike trail. If you have not seen this part of

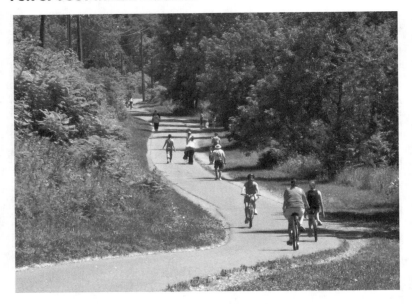

The Popular Shared-Use Trail North of Downtown

the world before, follow the trail a short distance to the right to Charlie's Boat House, where there are seasonal restrooms and snacks. A little further on is the recently finished trail bridge across the Winooski River. This is an exciting development, since it signals the start of the Island Line trail northward. However, today, there is not much that way for the on-footer, unless you are seeking a lengthy out-and-back run.

Head south on the Lake Champlain Path, noting the seven-mile marker here. On a nice day, expect many other trail users—both cyclists and pedestrians.

Cross Starr Farm Road, Stanford Road, and Shore Road. Then pass the Leddy Park Arena access road. One mile after Leddy Park you reach North Beach. This is a very pleasant and popular beach, with restrooms and a kiosk open daily in summer. It is roughly two miles to downtown from here.

Continue to Waterfront Park. There is some risk of encountering crowds here, since it is the venue of several local festivals. You then come to the aquarium, where there are restrooms and a visitor information booth. If you would like more maps and more local trail information, continue one block further south to the Local Motion Trailside center.

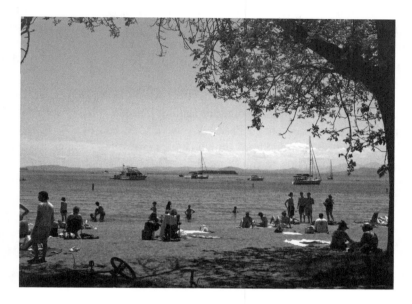

North Beach

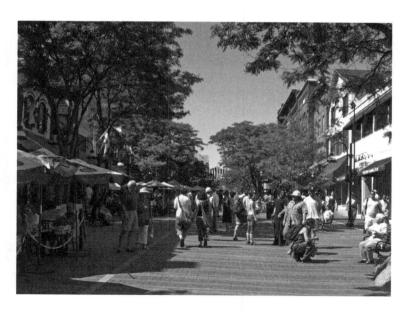

Colorful Church Street Marketplace

The aquarium, which is at College Street, is a good place to turn inland back to the center of downtown. Following College Street, pass the Vermont Pub and Brewery. This is an excellent pub and restaurant, with a menu including traditional English pub favorites (and real food too).

One block further on is Church Street Marketplace, a very lively pedestrian street with many outdoor seating places. It has a style and environment reminiscent of Paris. We have tried and like Ri Ra and Sweetwaters on Church Street, but you have many other choices around here for a post-exercise drink or meal.

Burlington: Ethan Allen Homestead

Distance	6.7 miles
Comfort	Roughly 3.8 miles on a paved multi-use trail, 0.9 miles on an unpaved pedestrian path, and a mile each way along street sidewalks getting to and from the trails. Expect ample other people near the two ends, but people may be sparse on the multi-use trail. Only the multi-use trail is suitable for inline skating.
Attractions	The Ethan Allen Homestead was the last home of the man who dominates early Vermont history. The restored home is open seasonally for tours (check opening hours in advance) and there is a small accompanying museum. There are also some attractive riverside pedestrian trails and elevated boardwalks through wetlands nearby. The multi-use trail between downtown and the Homestead is an excellent place for on-foot exercise, regardless of whether you want to stop to soak up history at the Homestead.
Convenience	Start and end near City Hall in downtown Burlington. If you are staying at one of the many hotels on Williston Road beyond the University, it is about 1.5 miles each way to/from downtown on-foot via a good sidewalk, or there is a bus service.
Destination	Downtown Burlington's Church Street Market-place, with its many shops, restaurants, and pubs.

This route is less a single canned formula than a collection of ideas you can adapt in various ways to suit your own tastes. If you are interested in a straightforward run or jog, with minimal interference from traffic, focus on the multi-use trail to the Homestead and beyond. You can also tack on some peaceful pedestrian trail loops near the Homestead. If you are mainly interested in seeing the Homestead, consider making some use of the trails mentioned, as a way of gaining some fitness as well as history knowledge.

You can start virtually anywhere downtown; we chose to start in Church Street near City Hall. Go north through Church Street

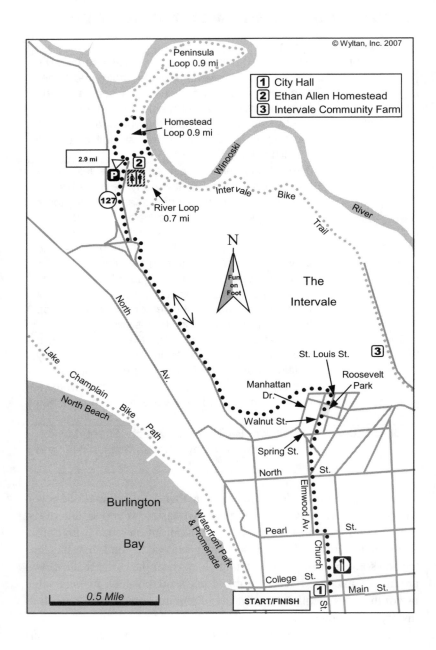

© Wyltan, Inc. 2007

Peninsula
Loop 0.9 mi

1	City Hall
2	Ethan Allen Homestead
3	Intervale Community Farm

Homestead
Loop 0.9 mi

2.9 mi

127

River Loop
0.7 mi

Winooski

Intervale Bike Trail

River

N

Fun
on
Foot

The

Intervale

St. Louis St.

3

North

Roosevelt
Park

Manhattan
Dr.

Lake Champlain Bike Path

North Beach

Walnut St.

Spring St.

North St.

Av.

Elmwood Av.

Burlington

Waterfront Park & Promenade

Pearl St.

Bay

Church St.

College St.

0.5 Mile

START/FINISH

1

Main St.

Marketplace to Pearl Street. Do a left-then-right dogleg here into Elmwood Avenue. Follow Elmwood to its end and then bear right into Walnut Street, following it one block to the small park, Roosevelt Park. Go around or through the park to Saint Louis Street, heading north. At the intersection of Saint Louis with Manhattan Drive you find the trailhead for the paved multi-use trail that takes you to Ethan Allen Homestead.

Saint Louis Street and the start of the trail are not in the best part of town, but that situation improves when you get onto the trail proper. It is quite pleasant, has a good paved surface, and you should expect to pass the occasional other trail user. However, I would caution that this is one trail you might feel more comfortable with if you have a companion.

The trail tracks the edge of the highway, Route 127. Continue to where the trail diverts around a highway exit ramp. Follow the trail as it turns to the right, along the access road to Ethan Allen Homestead. Pass a trailhead for the River Loop—this is a low trail hugging a wetlands area and may be impassable depending on the season and recent weather.

If you keep to the paved trail, it leads to the 1787-vintage Homestead and its adjacent museum. When Nola and I were last there, the museum was open and its enthusiastic volunteers were offering tours of the Homestead. It was well worth taking the time to do the tour.

At this point, you have a choice of unpaved on-foot trails you might wish to traverse. The one that we have included in the featured route is called the Homestead Loop, a 0.9-mile loop around the scenic river plains near the Homestead. If you take this loop, you have the option of also adding on the Peninsula Loop, down the river from the Homestead. If you do that, it adds 1.5 miles to your distance.

When you have experienced enough of the Homestead area, retrace your steps back along the multi-use trail to downtown Burlington. By then, you will likely be ready for a wind-down drink or snack in Church Street Marketplace.

VARIATION

There is an alternate route back to downtown via the Intervale Bike Trail (see our map). While this offers a pleasant escape from traffic and people, be warned however that the underfoot conditions are highly variable and the end part of the trail near and after the community farm traverses a far-less-than-beautiful industrial area.

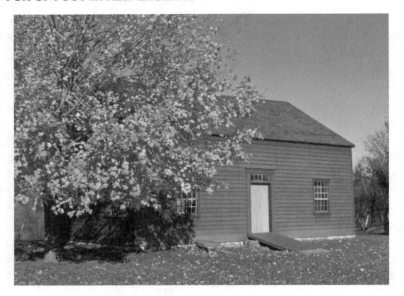

Ethan Allen Homestead (1787)

Montpelier: Hubbard Park Short Loop

Distance	2.4 miles
Comfort	Follow quiet, pedestrian-friendly sidewalks for 1.7 miles, with the remaining 0.7 miles on pleasant pedestrian trails in a wooded park. There are some significant grades, but a fit person can easily run the entire route. Expect plenty of other people around, mostly relaxed locals, but no crowds. Not suitable for inline skating.
Attractions	The natural beauty of Montpelier and Hubbard Park. Pass the majestic Vermont State House.
Convenience	Start and end near the post office in State Street, in the center of Montpelier.
Destination	The center of Montpelier, with its shops and a selection of local restaurants.

Despite the prestigious role of the state capital of Vermont, Montpelier has the demeanor of a lovely little country town. With a population around the 8,000 mark, Montpelier is no metropolis. The attitudes of the locals reflect this. It is a very friendly place. Everyone exchanges greetings on the street. Everyone looks relaxed. Motorists treat pedestrians like royalty—the pedestrian always has the right of way. On one occasion I moved close to the curb taking photos and was surprised to find the drivers stopping, thinking that maybe I was about to cross the street.

Montpelier also has some outstanding on-foot exercise places very close to its center, so there is no excuse for being unfit here. We have documented two Montpelier routes—a short but sweet one into the city's Hubbard Park, and a slightly longer one that extends from Hubbard Park into North Branch Park.

From the city's heart by the post office in State Street, follow Elm Street eastward. Turn left into Spring Street. At the end of the street, go straight ahead into Parkway Avenue, a narrow one-way street, but cars are so sparse they are unlikely to worry you. Proceed up the hill into Hubbard Park. You come to Frog Pond, where there is a parking area. I did not hear any frogs but it is a lovely little pond and I have no doubt that frogs are there.

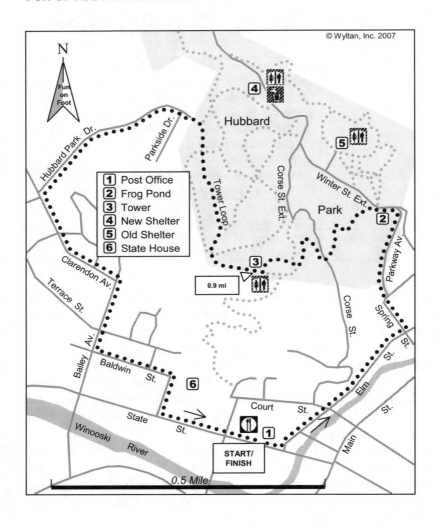

© Wyltan, Inc. 2007

From Frog Pond take the footpath up the hill to the left. This path weaves up the hill to an old road, which is an extension of Corse Street. Cross the road and continue up the weaving trail to the 54-foot stone observation tower. You can climb the 65 steps to the top of the tower, where you can see a long way, but in summer the view consists almost entirely of green trees. There is a restroom here.

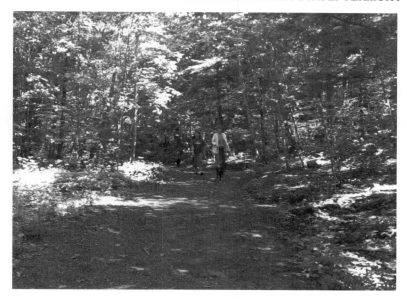

A Typically Leafy Hubbard Park Trail

VARIATION
   There is a somewhat steep path from the tower down to Court Street, not far from the State House. You might choose to build this into your exercise route if steepness does not bother you.

While there are different ways back to town from here, we suggest following the Tower Loop westward—this was once a road but is now car-less and excellent for running. Continue to the Hubbard Park Drive gate, which is now permanently closed.

Exit the park via that gate and follow Hubbard Park Drive downhill. Go left into Clarendon Avenue and then right into Bailey Avenue. Then turn left into Baldwin Street, which takes you to the State House. This is a really beautiful State House, complete with a gold leaf dome, and a park with colorful gardens in front.

The State House fronts onto State Street. Follow State Street a couple of blocks downhill to the post office where we started.

If you want a wind-down snack or drink, there are not many choices. We can personally recommend Julio's Cantina in State Street, and we hear that McGillicuddy's Irish Pub at Langdon Street and Main Street is also a great place.

Montpelier: Hubbard and North Branch Parks

Distance	3.7 miles
Comfort	Follow pedestrian-friendly sidewalks for 1.8 miles, with the remaining 1.9 miles on pleasant pedestrian trails in wooded parks. There are some significant grades, but a fit person can easily run the entire route. Expect plenty of other people around, mostly relaxed locals, but no crowds. Not suitable for inline skating.
Attractions	The natural beauty of Montpelier and its two parks, Hubbard Park and North Branch Park.
Convenience	Start and end near the post office in State Street, in the center of Montpelier.
Destination	The center of Montpelier, with its shops and a selection of local restaurants.

Our second Montpelier route builds on the first one, taking in some more of Hubbard Park and also part of Montpelier's other major park, North Branch Park.

As in our previous route, start by the post office in State Street and follow Elm Street eastward. Turn left into Spring Street. At the end of the street, go straight ahead into Parkway Avenue. Proceed up the hill to Frog Pond.

You now need to get to the New Shelter. There are several ways to do that, including the main road, the path via the Old Shelter called the Fitness Trail, and the trail via the observation tower that we followed in the previous route. For mileage purposes, we assume the latter. From Frog Pond take the footpath up the hill to the left. Cross the extension of Corse Street and continue up to the observation tower. Follow Tower Loop to the west and north, to the Hubbard Park Drive gate. Pass that gate and continue on the trail to the New Shelter.

Continue up the road called 7 Fireplaces Way. At the end of the road there are restrooms and—you guessed it—seven fireplaces.

From here, pick up the foot trail heading north. Follow the sign to Parks Connector, which is the trail linking Hubbard Park to North Branch Park.

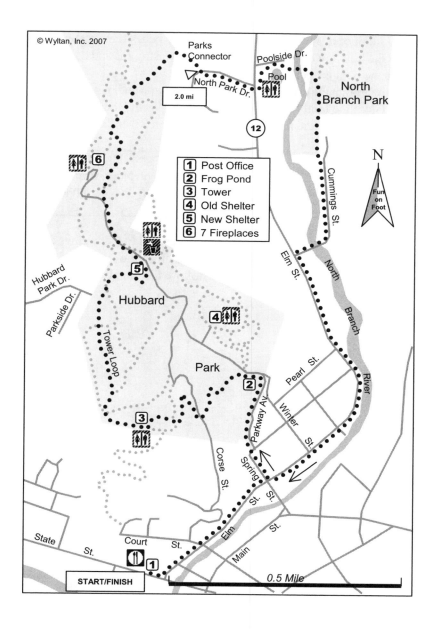

© Wyltan, Inc. 2007

Parks Connector

Poolside Dr.

Pool

North Branch Park

North Park Dr.

2.0 mi

12

1	Post Office
2	Frog Pond
3	Tower
4	Old Shelter
5	New Shelter
6	7 Fireplaces

6

Cummings St.

N

Fun on Foot

Elm St.

North Branch

5

Hubbard

Hubbard Park Dr.

Parkside Dr.

Tower Loop

4

Old Shelter

Park

2

Pearl St.

Winter

River

Parkway Av.

St.

3

Corse St.

Spring

St.

St.

State St.

Court

St.

Elm

Main

0.5 Mile

1

START/FINISH

The Parks Connector trail ends at North Park Drive. Follow this street to Route 12. Cross Route 12 at the pedestrian crossing (being thankful once again that cars always stop for pedestrians around here). Take the trail down past the pool. There are restrooms and a kiosk here when the pool is open.

Go through the car park, with the tennis courts and ball field on your left. Cross the footbridge over the river into North Branch Park. Bear towards the right and pick up the North Branch River Park Trail.

VARIATION

There are some pleasant foot trails through North Branch Park, heading north and east from our route. You can tack on a mile or so here if you wish.

The North Branch River Park Trail takes you to Cummings Street. Follow quiet Cummings Street south and cross the river on the road bridge. Go left into Elm Street and follow the sidewalk back to the center of town.

Other Routes

Vermont offers many opportunities for outdoor exercise but, since the state is somewhat short of cities and large towns, there is not a lot that fits the model for this book.

The largest population center of Vermont is **Greater Burlington**, including the cities or towns of **South Burlington**, **Winooski**, and **Colchester**. Roughly a quarter of the population of the state lives here. We covered two routes, convenient to downtown Burlington. Here are some ideas for other routes in the region...

The **Lake Champlain Bike Path** extends both south and north of the first route we described in this chapter. You can follow the trail south along the lakeshore roughly 2.5 miles to Oakledge Park. There is a bus service back to downtown should you need that. Another possibility here is to head inland along Home Avenue on street sidewalks, cross Route 7, and pick up the paved multi-use trail east and north to the University of Vermont campus. This might work for you if you are staying in one of the Williston Road hotels.

The Lake Champlain Bike Path continues north of the trail bridge over the Winooski River, roughly five miles along the old rail causeway (Causeway Park) to a break in the causeway. There are plans for a bike and pedestrian ferry across the break, which will give access to the South Hero island community. While attractive for cyclists, this is unlikely to prove an exciting route for any but the hardiest on-footer.

Roughly six miles south of downtown Burlington is **Shelburne Bay**, which has some attractive pedestrian trails in both Shelburne Bay Park and in the Shelburne Farms area.

At **Malletts Bay** in **Colchester**, about five miles north of downtown Burlington, there are good on-foot exercise opportunities both along the lakeshore and on the Colchester Bike Path.

Roughly 30 miles north of Greater Burlington is the city of Saint Albans and the start of the **Missisquoi Valley Rail Trail**. This 26-mile gravel trail traverses Sheldon Springs, Sheldon Junction, North Sheldon, South Franklin, Enosburg Falls, and North Enosburg, ending in Richford.

There are innumerable excellent hiking trails in Vermont. There are over 50 state parks, most of which have pedestrian trails, but they are not generally close to population centers. If you are a very serious hiker, you should also consider the Appalachian Trail, which extends from the southwest corner of Vermont to the Connecticut River at Hanover, New Hampshire, and the Long Trail from Killington in the south to the Canadian border in the north.

* * * *

Vermont, with its mountains, woods, and placid lifestyle, is an excellent place for outdoor exercise in summer and winter alike. Enjoy the Green Mountain State!

11

Conclusion

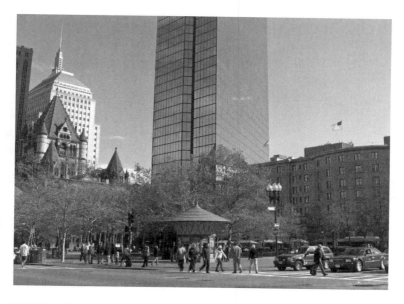

The Boston Marathon ends in Copley Square (photo above).
What more appropriate image could we use to end our book?
Nola and I have enormously enjoyed collecting the material for
this manuscript. We thought we already knew New England quite well,
having lived in the region ten years, but we learnt an enormous amount
more during our research on this book.

We know we have only scratched the surface in documenting the
best places to run, jog, or walk in New England. Nevertheless, we hope
that our approach of focusing on the larger cities and the places that
attract most visitors will provide the most benefit to people seeking
motivating ideas for spending more time outdoors on foot.

FUN OF FOOT IN NEW ENGLAND

There is no doubt that New England is an excellent place for outdoor exercise, and we encourage all readers to build their own favorite routes using the ideas in this book plus ideas of their own.

Enjoy New England and keep fit!

Index

A

Acadia National Park 200
Amherst 148
Appalachian Trail 236, 278
Arlington 66, 89
Arnold Arboretum 37
Ashuelot Rail Trail 234
attractions 4
Auburn ME 201
Augusta 195

B

Back Bay 15, 22, 55
Back Bay Fens 34
Back Cove 185
Bangor 201
Bar Harbor 200
Barnstable 119
Barrington 250
Bay Circuit Trail 148
Beacon Hill 46
Benton 202
Bethel ME 201
Beverly 90
Blackstone River Bikeway 148,
   258
Blue Hills Reservation 89
Boothbay Harbor 201
Boston 11, 15, 32
Boston Common 24, 32
Boston Marathon 55
Boston Public Garden 23
Boston University (BU) 18
Bretton Woods 235
Brewster 97
Bridgeport 177
Bristol 248

Brookline 32, 35, 55
Brown University 239
Brunswick ME 201
BU Bridge 18
Burlington 262, 267
Buzzards Bay 119

C

calories burned 5
Cambridge 15, 40, 61, 66
Camden 201
Cape Cod 91
Cape Cod Canal 119
Cape Cod Rail Trail 97
Cape Elizabeth 200
Cape Poge Wildlife Refuge 110
Carrabassett Valley 201
Castle Island 29
Chappaquiddick 110
Charles River 15, 25, 61
Charles River mileages 25
Chatham 97, 119
Cheshire Branch Rail Trail 234
Chestnut Hill Reservoir 46, 59
Chicopee 148
Cliff Walk 252
Cohasset 89
Colchester 277
comfort 3
Commonwealth Avenue 22, 32, 34
Concord MA 130
Concord NH 214, 217, 234
Connecticut River Walk and Bike-
   way 148
convenience 4
Copley Square 59
Cove Island Park 173
crime indexes 9
Cumberland 258
Cummings Park 173

FUN ON FOOT

in America's Cities

By Warwick Ford
with Nola Ford

Where to run, jog, walk in...

Atlanta • Boston • Chicago • Dallas • Denver
Indianapolis • Los Angeles • Minneapolis
New York • Philadelphia • San Diego
San Francisco • Seattle • Washington

The book featured in *USA Today* and *Los Angeles Times*

Highly recommended for all public libraries in the states in which the aforementioned cities are located and for large public libraries throughout the rest of the country. **Library Journal**

Fun on Foot in America's Cities ... is the ultimate guide to the "unseen" America via foot travel. *Fun on Foot* is very highly recommended to all American vacationers, especially those in-tune with nature.
The Midwest Book Review

As an avid jogger and well-traveled executive of a California telecom firm, Warwick Ford could write a book on great places to run in big cities across the USA. And now he has...
USA Today

It's a fitness plan so simple it's stunning. So simple, in fact, it's disguised as a guide book. *Fun on Foot* resonated with me instantly. ... In a very real way, *Fun on Foot* is a guide book, but it's also much more.
January Magazine

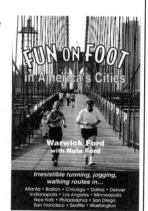

Wyltan Books   Paper, 388 pp   190 illustrations
ISBN 978-0-9765244-0-3   (ISBN-10: 0-9765244-0-6)

About the Authors

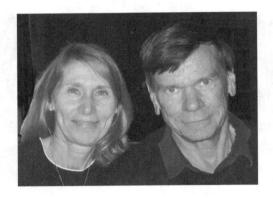

Warwick Ford and Nola Ford are Australian-raised Canadian-Americans with a passion for running, skiing, and travel. As a Massachusetts-based executive of a California company, Warwick spent years as a road warrior, bunking down in different cities. One of the biggest challenges of that period was finding the motivation and the time to get out on foot enough to maintain fitness. That led to the book *Fun on Foot in America's Cities*, which packages for travelers the very best on-foot exercise routes in 14 major cities. Now, with Nola's collusion, Warwick has applied the same model to their home region, New England. Warwick's educational qualifications include a Ph. D. from the University of Toronto. In his earlier life, he authored technical books including *Computer Communications Security* and *Secure Electronic Commerce*.